POCKET GUIDE TO
NURSING DIAGNOSES

POCKET GUIDE TO
NURSING
DIAGNOSES

FIFTH EDITION

Mi Ja Kim, RN, PhD, FAAN
Professor and Dean
College of Nursing
University of Illinois at Chicago
Chicago, Illinois

Gertrude K. McFarland, RN, DNSc, FAAN
Health Scientist Administrator
Nursing Research Study Section
Division of Research Grants
National Institutes of Health, USPHS
U.S. Department of Health and Human Services
Bethesda, Maryland

Audrey M. McLane, RN, PhD
Professor Emerita
College of Nursing
Marquette University
Milwaukee, Wisconsin

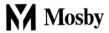 Mosby

St. Louis Baltimore Boston Chicago London Philadelphia Sydney Toronto

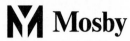

Mosby

Dedicated to Publishing Excellence

Publisher: Alison Miller
Editor: Terry Van Schaik
Developmental Editor: Janet Livingston
Project Manager: Carol Sullivan Wiseman
Senior Production Editor: David S. Brown
Senior Designer: Jeanne Wolfgeher

FIFTH EDITION

Printed in the United States of America

Mosby–Year Book, Inc.
11830 Westline Industrial Drive, St. Louis, Missouri 63146

Library of Congress Cataloging in Publication Data

Pocket guide to nursing diagnoses / [edited by] Mi Ja Kim, Gertrude
  K. McFarland, Audrey M. McLane.   5th ed.
        p.   cm.
  Includes bibliographical references and index.
  ISBN 0-8016-6669-4
  1. Nursing diagnosis.   I. Kim, Mi Ja.   II. McFarland, Gertrude
K., 1941.   III. McLane, Audrey M.
  [DNLM: 1. Nursing Diagnosis—handbooks.   2. Patient Care
  Planning—handbooks.   WY 39 P739]
RT48.6.P63 1993
616.07'5   dc20
DNLM/DLC
for Library of Congress   92-48806
                                                              CIP

93   94   95   96   97   GW/DC   9   8   7   6   5   4   3   2   1

CONTRIBUTORS

Kim Astroth, RN, MS
Instructor
Mennonite College of Nursing
Bloomington, Illinois

Sarah McNabb Badalamenti, RN, MSN
Clinical Nurse Specialist
St. Joseph's Hospital
Milwaukee, Wisconsin

Thelma I. Bates, RN, MSN, CS
Psychiatric Clinical Specialist
Washington Hospital Center
Washington, DC

Joan M. Caley, RN, MS, CS, CNAA*
Associate Chief, Nursing Service
V.A. Medical Center
Portland, Oregon

Nancy S. Creason, BSN, MSN, PhD
Professor and Dean, School of Nursing
Southern Illinois University at Edwardsville
Edwardsville, Illinois

Kathryn T. Czurylo, RN, MS, CS
Surgical Clinical Nurse Specialist
Alexian Brothers Medical Center
Elk Grove Village, Illinois

Donna M. Dixon, RN, MS
Educational Coordinator
Department of Nursing Education and Research
Children's Memorial Medical Center
Chicago, Illinois

*The opinions expressed herein are those of the authors and do not necessarily reflect those of the National Institutes of Health, U.S. Public Health Service, U.S. Department of Health and Human Services, the Veterans Administration, or the Uniformed Services University of the Health Sciences.

CONTRIBUTORS

Susan Dudas, RN, MSN, FAAN
Associate Professor
College of Nursing
University of Illinois at Chicago
Chicago, Illinois

Teresa L. Fadden, RN, MSN, CS
Clinical Nurse IV
St. Joseph's Hospital
Milwaukee, Wisconsin

Richard J. Fehring, RN, DNSc
Associate Professor
Marquette University College of Nursing
Milwaukee, Wisconsin

Margaret I. Fitch, RN, PhD
Oncology Nurse Researcher, Comprehensive Cancer Program
Toronto-Bayview Regional Cancer Center/
Sunnybrook Health Science Center
North York, Ontario, Canada

Michele C. Gattuso, RN, MS
Clinical Nurse Specialist/Maternal Child Health
Alexian Brothers Medical Center
Elk Grove Village, Illinois

Elizabeth Kelchner Gerety, RN, MS, CS, FAAN*
Clinical Nurse Specialist
Psychiatry Consultation
Portland Veterans Affairs Medical Center
Portland, Oregon

Jane E. Graydon, BScN, MS, PhD
Associate Professor
Faculty of Nursing
University of Toronto
Toronto, Ontario, Canada

Mary V. Hanley, RN, MA*
Critical Care Instructor, Nursing Education
Veterans Affairs Medical Center/Outpatient Clinics
Boston, Massachusetts

Marilyn Harter, RN, MSN, CRRN
Clinical Nurse Specialist
Rehabilitation and Neurology
Columbia Hospital
Milwaukee, Wisconsin

Kathryn Hennessy, RN, MS, CNSN
Clinical Nursing Manager/Nutrition Support Nurse
Caremark Healthcare Services
Lincolnshire, Illinois

Pamela D. Hill, RN, BSN, MS, PhD
Assistant Professor
Department of Maternal Child Nursing
College of Nursing, Quad-Cities Regional Site
University of Illinois
Rock Island, Illinois

Karen Inaba, MS, RN, CS, PMHNP
Psychiatric Consultation-Liaison Clinical Nurse Specialist
University Hospital
Assistant Professor
Department of Mental Health Nursing
Oregon Health Sciences University
Portland, Oregon

Joyce H. Johnson, RN, BSN, MSN, PhD
Associate Professor
College of Nursing
University of Illinois at Chicago
Chicago, Illinois

Karen Kavanaugh, RN, PhD
Assistant Professor
College of Nursing
University of Illinois at Chicago
Chicago, Illinois

Jin H. Kim, RN, MSN
Doctoral Student
College of Nursing
University of Illinois at Chicago
Chicago, Illinois

CONTRIBUTORS

Mi Ja Kim, RN, PhD, FAAN
Professor and Dean
College of Nursing
University of Illinois at Chicago
Chicago, Illinois

Pamela Wolfe Kohlbry, RN, MSN
Camarillo, California

Patricia A. Koller, RN, MSN
Clinical Care Nurse III, Intensive Care
St. Joseph's Hospital
Milwaukee, Wisconsin

Carol E. Kupperberg, RN, MSN
Home Care Case Manager
Children's Home Health Care Services
Children's National Medical Center
Washington, DC

Jane Lancour, MSN, RN
Associate Administrator
Director of Nursing
FHP Hospital
Fountain Valley, California

Janet L. Larson, RN, PhD
Associate Professor
College of Nursing
University of Illinois at Chicago
Chicago, Illinois

Lorna A. Larson, BA, BS, MSN, DNSc
Ft. Washington, Maryland

Marie Maguire, RN, MSN
Clinical Nurse Specialist
Lakeland Nursing Home of Wallworth County
Elkhorn, Wisconsin

Mary E. Markert, RN, MN
Acting Branch Chief, Geropsychiatry
DC Commission on Mental Health Services
Washington, DC

Gertrude K. McFarland, RN, DNSc, FAAN*
Health Scientist Administrator
Nursing Research Study Section
Division of Research Grants
National Institutes of Health, USPHS
U.S. Department of Health and Human Services
Bethesda, Maryland

Audrey M. McLane, RN, PhD
Professor Emerita
College of Nursing
Marquette University
Milwaukee, Wisconsin

Ruth E. McShane, RN, PhD
Assistant Professor
School of Nursing
University of Wisconsin-Milwaukee
Milwaukee, Wisconsin

Judy Minton, RNC, MS
Nurse Practitioner
Decatur, Illinois

Victoria L. Mock, RN, DNSc, OCN
Assistant Professor
Boston College School of Nursing
Boston, Massachusetts

Martha M. Morris, RN, EdD
Director, BSN Program
Maryville University
St. Louis, Missouri

Charlotte E. Naschinski, RN, AAS, BSN, MS*
Deputy Director, Continuing Health Professional Education
Uniformed Services University of the Health Sciences
Bethesda, Maryland

Emma B. Nemivant, RN, BSN, MED, MSN
Clinical Instructor
College of Nursing
University of Illinois at Chicago
Chicago, Illinois

CONTRIBUTORS

Colleen M. O'Brien, RN, MSN, CCRN
Educator–Critical and Intermediate Care
Bellin Hospital
Green Bay, Wisconsin

Linda O'Brien-Pallas, RN, PhD
Assistant Professor and Career Scientist
Director, Quality of Worklife Research Unit
Faculty of Nursing
University of Toronto
Toronto, Ontario, Canada

Annette M. O'Connor, RN, PhD
Professor
School of Nursing
University of Ottawa
Ottawa, Ontario, Canada

Sheila Olson, RN, MSN
Onalaska, Wisconsin

Catherine J. Ryan, RN, MS, CCRN
Clinical Nurse Specialist-Critical Care
Alexian Brothers Medical Center
Elk Grove Village, Illinois

Karen V. Scipio-Skinner, RN, MSN
Legislative/Practice Specialist
DC Nurses Association
Washington, DC

Maureen E. Shekleton, BSN, MSN, DNSc
Adjunct Assistant Professor, Medical-Surgical Nursing
University of Illinois at Chicago
Chicago, Illinois

Kathleen C. Sheppard, RN, PhD
Director of Nursing, Continuity of Care
University of Texas
M.D. Anderson Cancer Center
Houston, Texas

Margaret J. Stafford, RN, MSN, FAAN
Associate Professor
College of Nursing
University of Illinois at Chicago
Chicago, Illinois

Janet F. Stansberry, RN, MSN
Clinical Nurse Specialist, Infertility
University of Pennsylvania
Philadelphia, Pennsylvania

Rosemarie Suhayda, RN, PhD
Assistant Professor
Rush University College of Nursing
Chicago, Illinois

Alice M. Tse, RN, PhD
University of Hawaii at Manoa
School of Nursing
Honolulu, Hawaii

Evelyn L. Wasli, RN, DNSc
Chief Nurse
Emergency Psychiatric Response Division
DC Commission on Mental Health Service
Washington, DC

Linda K. Young, RN, MSN
Nursing Faculty
Milwaukee County Medical Complex
School of Nursing
Milwaukee, Wisconsin

NANDA's Working Definition of Nursing Diagnosis

Nursing Diagnosis is a clinical judgment about individual, family, or community responses to actual or potential health problems/life processes. Nursing diagnoses provide the basis for selection of nursing interventions to achieve outcomes for which the nurse is accountable.

Approved at the Ninth Conference on Classification of Nursing Diagnoses.

PREFACE

Since the first edition of the *Pocket Guide to Nursing Diagnoses*, nursing diagnoses have become integrated into nursing education, research, and practice in the United States. In addition, nursing diagnosis has gained acceptance in countries such as Canada, France, The Netherlands, Australia, Italy, Taiwan, Spain, Slovenia, Denmark, Korea, and other countries. Nursing students find nursing diagnoses to be a useful tool of learning. Both nursing students and practicing nurses find nursing diagnoses a useful way of conceptualizing nursing science and focusing for clinical decision making. Educators have adopted nursing diagnoses as an organizing framework for teaching and practice. Nurse researchers are using nursing diagnoses as a focus for research while the NANDA Taxonomy taken as a whole presents a challenge for systematic validation through research. The nursing profession and its specialty organizations recognize the contribution of a nursing nosology to their ability to demonstrate the effectiveness of nursing practice and to influence health care policy.

The major purposes of the *Pocket Guide* continue to be:
1. to present the most up-to-date information on NANDA nursing diagnoses terminology, definitions, related/risk/contextual factors, and defining characteristics
2. to present a prototype state-of-the-art care plan for each nursing diagnosis
3. to provide an easy-to-use guide for clinicians, faculty, and students in their daily practice
4. to stimulate critical thinking of practical nurses, and
5. to facilitate the use of theory and research-based nursing interventions in the practice setting.

We are deeply indebted to the users of this book who generously provided their suggestions and who continue to endorse this book.

In keeping with the philosophy of the previous editions, every effort has been made to make this *Pocket Guide* easy to use while providing a theoretical and research base for each prototype care plan. We have chosen to present nursing diagnoses in alphabetical order because the conceptual framework for the organization of nursing diagnoses is still under development. The current NANDA Taxonomy I Revised 1992 version is presented in Appendix A for those who may want to know the taxonomic structure for these diagnoses.

The senior authors have added 10 new nursing diagnoses that were approved by NANDA members following the Tenth Conference on Classification of Nursing Diagnoses in San Diego, California in 1992. These diagnoses are Caregiver Role Strain, Dysfunctional Ventilatory Weaning Response, High Risk for Caregiver Role Strain, High Risk for Peripheral Neurovascular Dysfunction, High Risk for Self-Mutilation, Inability to Sustain Spontaneous Ventilation, Ineffective Infant Feeding Pattern, Ineffective Management of Therapeutic Regimen, Interrupted Breastfeeding, and Relocation Stress Syndrome.

Defining characteristics and related/risk factors presented are NANDA approved, and the same is true for the majority of definitions. Definitions of nursing diagnoses approved by NANDA have been used to the extent they were developed. For completeness, we developed definitions for diagnoses that do not have definitions.

A concerted effort has been made to present nursing care plans as prototypes rather than standard care plans. By making the care plans prototypes, we have emphasized that they are for specific individuals or a group of patients with specified related/risk factors. Therefore in applying these plans to patients, practicing nurses will need to give specific consideration to individual patient requirements. Acuity and severity of nursing diagnoses are other dimensions that were not addressed in these care plans for the sake of brevity. These are other important factors for nurses to consider when individualizing these care plans.

Each care plan was developed on the basis of a nursing diagnosis that comprises a diagnostic label and the term *related to* for related or risk factors. For example, if the nursing diagnosis is High Risk for Injury with a risk factor of "emotional lability," the nurse would record this as "High risk for injury related to emotional lability." We used the following guide for the development of the prototype care plans.

- The patient goals/expected outcomes reflect the desired health state of a patient and specify indicators addressing the extent of achievement of the patient goal(s).
- Scientific rationale are specified for interventions or cluster of interventions.
- Patient conditions are specified where the care plan is more focused for a specific type of patient.
- Nursing interventions are selected to address related factors or risk factors, to ameliorate/modify defining characteristics, and to assist patients in achieving their goals and optimal health state.

The care plans were developed from a perspective of persons interacting with their environment in the pursuit of health. The use of nursing diagnoses and relevant nursing interventions that are designed to meet patient goals has sharpened the focus of current practice and has demonstrated the potential of nursing diagnoses for contributing to quality health care.

Contributing authors of the *Pocket Guide* are clinical experts who reflect the state-of-the-art and science of nursing practice. We acknowledge substantive contributions made by practicing nurses to the development and refinement of nursing diagnoses. Practicing nurses are encouraged to engage in critical thinking while using the prototype care plans. Their participation in research on all nursing diagnoses is essential for the national and international development of nursing diagnoses taxonomy and a scientific base for nursing practice. There is a critical need to comprehensively evaluate the nursing diagnostic terminology and taxonomy through on-going nursing research.

Mi Ja Kim
Gertrude K. McFarland
Audrey M. McLane

USING THE POCKET GUIDE TO NURSING DIAGNOSES

Pattern recognition, validation of judgments, and interpretation of clinical meaning within a particular context are basic cognitive skills registered nurses bring to a patient/family health care situation. Pattern recognition in response to cues (defining characteristics) may occur at any point in the assessment process. Assessment data may be gathered to facilitate pattern recognition and/or validate the existence of a previously recognized pattern.

Subjective and objective assessment data are gathered with respect to a presenting situation or longer-term health status, activities and demands of daily living, and internal and external resources (current and potential) of a patient/family. Nursing diagnoses, agreed-on labels for diagnostic concepts, are assigned to recognized patterns. A nursing diagnosis for a patient/family health care situation includes a diagnostic label and related factors contributing to the onset/maintenance of an actual diagnosis or a diagnostic label and risk factors of a high risk diagnosis. Validation and interpretation of a diagnosis and related/risk factors are ongoing processes of cue recognition and pattern recognition. A nursing diagnosis, then, becomes the focal point for developing goals, expected outcomes, interventions, and evaluation.

SECTION ONE

Diagnostic terminology, definitions, related/risk/contextual factors, and defining characteristics for NANDA-approved diagnoses are included in Section One of the *Pocket Guide to Nursing Diagnoses*. Each diagnosis has a set of components: definition, defining characteristics, and related/contextual factors or definition and risk factors that are useful in several stages of the diagnostic process. A definition is a conceptual aid to understanding the meaning of a diagnostic term (Gordon, 1987). Defining characteristics that form a pattern help to operationalize the meaning within a particular context. Risk/related factors are patient behaviors and elements in the environment that interact to place an individual at high risk of developing a diagnosis or have contributed to the onset or maintenance of an actual diagnosis.

During an initial assessment, a nurse may develop a hypothesis on the basis of one or two cues (defining characteristics). The definition of a diagnosis and a pattern of defining characteristics could guide a search for additional signs/symptoms and help differentiate closely related diagnoses. The presence or absence of one or more related/risk factors helps to establish the status of a diagnosis, actual or high risk.

Writing a diagnostic statement and comparing it with a NANDA listing for the diagnosis provides intellectual stimuli for data analysis and a clinical decision. Comparison and validation increase confidence in the diagnosis and enable the nurse to proceed with setting goals, expected outcomes, and interventions.

SECTION TWO

Prototype care plans for all NANDA-approved diagnoses are included in Section Two of the *Pocket Guide to Nursing Diagnoses*. A prototype is a model or exemplar that demonstrates how the scientific knowledge embedded in a diagnosis can be used in a particular situation. Exemplars contribute to the assimilation of a way of viewing patient care situations. The prototype care plans demonstrate the linkages among nursing diagnosis, interventions, and goals/expected outcomes. Expected outcomes operationalize goals that are, by comparison. more conceptual. Patient outcomes that are sensitive to nursing care must be identified before interventions are selected. A nursing intervention is defined as "any direct care treatment that a nurse performs on behalf of a client" (Bulechek and McCloskey, 1989, p. 25). An intervention may be implemented in a variety of ways. The nurse's understanding of the scientific rationale underlying the intervention and prior experience in treating a given diagnosis influence patient outcomes, i.e., successful treatment of the nursing diagnosis.

Scientific rationale are included in the prototype care plans in Section Two for nursing interventions. As scientific understanding of the mechanism(s) influencing the development/maintenance of a nursing diagnosis increases, new interventions may replace or may be used in addition to existing nursing interventions. Student nurses and nursing instructors may wish to elaborate on a scientific rationale or consider treatment alternatives to further a student's learning. Experienced nurses will know which interventions have been successful in a particular context. The prototype care plans demonstrate the product of clinical decision making. Because most patients will have more than one nursing diagnosis, priorities must be set, and acuity and severity of all diagnoses must be considered for nursing interventions. An intervention for one diagnosis may require modification because of the existence of other diagnoses.

The reference for a prototype care plan are numbered and placed at the bottom of the first page of each care plan. Nurses and students are encouraged to use the references as a resource to increase their understanding of the conceptual and scientific bases for the diagnoses.

SECTION THREE

NANDA's "to be developed" diagnostic concepts and definitions (TBDs) are included in Section Three of the *Pocket Guide to Nursing Diagnoses*. The components of TBDs are a diagnostic label and a definition. The "to be developed" category is used by NANDA to designate diagnoses that are partially developed and are deemed potentially useful to the profession. TBDs are included to stimulate further development and validation.

GLOSSARY

The definitions for terms listed in the glossary were prepared by the authors of the *Pocket Guide for Nursing Diagnoses*. They were included to clarify the meaning of selected terms used by the authors and contributors.

APPENDIXES

Appendix A is a classification of nursing diagnoses by human response patterns (NANDA Taxonomy I-revised 1992).

Appendix B is a classification of nursing diagnoses by functional health patterns (Gordon, 1993).

REFERENCES

Bulechek GM, McCloskey JC: Nursing interventions: treatments for nursing diagnoses. In Carroll-Johnson RM, ed: *Classification of nursing diagnoses: proceedings of the eighth conference*, Philadelphia, 1989, JB Lippincott.

Gordon M: *Nursing diagnosis: process and application*, ed 2, New York, 1987, McGraw-Hill.

Gordon M: *Manual of nursing diagnoses 1993-1994*, St Louis, 1993, Mosby–Year Book.

CONTENTS

Nursing diagnoses: definitions, related/risk factors, and defining characteristics

Activity intolerance
The state in which an individual has insufficient physiological or psychological energy to endure or complete required or desired daily activities.

Related factors
Generalized weakness
Sedentary life-style
Imbalance between oxygen supply and demand
Bed rest or immobility

Defining characteristics
Verbal report of fatigue or weakness
Abnormal heart rate or blood pressure response to activity
Exertional discomfort or dyspnea
Electrocardiographic changes reflecting arrhythmias or ischemia

Activity intolerance, potential
The state in which an individual is at risk of experiencing insufficient physiological or psychological energy to endure or complete required or desired daily activities.

Risk factors
History of previous intolerance
Deconditioned status
Presence of circulatory/respiratory problems
Inexperience with the activity

Adjustment, impaired
The state in which an individual is unable to modify his/her life-style/behavior in a manner consistent with a change in health status.

Related factors
Disability requiring change in life-style
Inadequate support systems
Impaired cognition
Sensory overload
Assault to self-esteem
Altered locus of control
Incomplete grieving

Defining characteristics
Verbalization of nonacceptance of health status change
Nonexistent or unsuccessful ability to be involved in problem solving or goal setting
Lack of movement toward independence

Extended period of shock, disbelief, or anger regarding health status change

Lack of future-oriented thinking

Airway clearance, ineffective
The state in which an individual is unable to clear secretions or obstructions from the respiratory tract to maintain airway patency.

Related factors
Decreased energy and fatigue

Tracheobronchial

    Infection

    Obstruction

    Secretion

Perceptual/cognitive impairment

Trauma

Defining characteristics
Abnormal breath sounds—rales (crackles), rhonchi (wheezes)

Changes in rate or depth of respiration

Tachypnea

Cough, effective or ineffective, with or without sputum

Cyanosis

Dyspnea

Fever

Anxiety
A vague, uneasy feeling, the source of which is often nonspecific or unknown to the individual.

Related factors
Unconscious conflict about essential values and goals of life

Threat to self-concept

Threat of death

Threat to or change in health status

Threat to or change in socioeconomic status

Threat to or change in role functioning

Threat to or change in environment

Threat to or change in interaction patterns

Situational and maturational crises

Interpersonal transmission and contagion

Unmet needs

Defining characteristics
Subjective

    Increased tension

    Apprehension

Increased helplessness
Uncertainty
Fear
Feeling of being scared
Feeling of inadequacy
Shakiness
Fear of unspecific consequences
Regretfulness
Overexcitedness
Feeling of being rattled
Distress
Jitteriness
Objective
Sympathetic stimulation—cardiovascular excitation, superficial vasoconstriction, pupil dilation
Restlessness
Insomnia
Glancing about
Poor eye contact
Trembling; hand tremors
Extraneous movements—foot shuffling; hand, arm movements
Expressed concern regarding changes in life events
Worry
Anxiety
Facial tension
Voice quivering
Focus on self
Increased wariness
Increased perspiration

Aspiration, high risk for
The state in which an individual is at risk for entry of gastric secretions, oropharyngeal secretions, or exogenous food or fluids into tracheobronchial passages due to dysfunction or absence of normal protective mechanisms.

Risk factors
Reduced level of consciousness
Depressed cough and gag reflexes
Presence of tracheotomy or endotracheal tube
Overinflated tracheotomy/endotracheal tube cuff
Inadequate tracheotomy/endotracheal tube cuff inflation

Gastrointestinal tubes
Bolus tube feedings/medication administration
Situations hindering elevation of upper body
Increased intragastric pressure
Increased gastric residual
Decreased gastrointestinal motility
Delayed gastric emptying
Impaired swallowing
Facial/oral/neck surgery or trauma
Wired jaws

Body image disturbance   Disruption in the way one perceives one's body image.

Related factors
Biophysical
Cognitive perceptual
Psychosocial
Cultural or spiritual

Defining characteristics
Either the following A or B must be present to justify the diagnosis of body image disturbance:

A. Verbal response to actual or perceived change in structure and/or function
B. Nonverbal response to actual or perceived change in structure and/or function

The following clinical manifestations may be used to validate the presence of A or B:

Objective
Missing body part
Actual change in structure and/or function
Not looking at body part
Not touching body part
Hiding or overexposing body part (intentional or unintentional)
Trauma to nonfunctioning part
Change in social involvement
Negative feelings about body
Feelings of helplessness, hopelessness, or powerlessness
Preoccupation with change or loss
Emphasis on remaining strengths, heightened achievement
Extension of body boundary to incorporate environmental objects

Personalization of part or loss by name
Depersonalization of part or loss by impersonal pronouns
Refusal to verify actual change

It may be possible to identify high-risk populations, such as those with the following conditions:

Missing body part
Dependence on a machine
Significance of body part or functioning with regard to age, gender, developmental level, or basic human needs
Physical change caused by biochemical agents (drugs)
Physical trauma or mutilation
Pregnancy and/or maturational changes

Body temperature, altered, high risk for The state in which an individual is at risk for failure to maintain body temperature within normal range.

Risk factors

Extremes of age
Extremes of weight
Exposure to cold/cool or warm/hot environments
Dehydration
Inactivity or vigorous activity
Medications causing vasoconstriction/vasodilation, altered metabolic rate, sedation
Inappropriate clothing for environmental temperature
Illness or trauma affecting temperature regulation

Bowel incontinence The state in which an individual experiences a change in normal bowel habits characterized by involuntary passage of stool.

Related factors

Neuromuscular involvement
Musculoskeletal involvement
Depression; severe anxiety
Perception or cognitive impairment

Defining characteristic

Involuntary passage of stool

Breastfeeding, effective The state in which a mother-infant dyad/family exhibits adequate proficiency and satisfaction with breastfeeding process.

Related factors

Basic breastfeeding knowledge

Normal breast structure
Normal infant oral structure
Infant gestational age greater than 34 weeks
Support sources
Maternal confidence

Defining characteristics

Mother able to position infant at breast to promote a successful latch-on response
Infant is content after feeding
Regular and sustained suckling/swallowing at the breast
Appropriate infant weight patterns for age
Effective mother-infant communication patterns (infant cues, maternal interpretation and response)
Signs and/or symptoms of oxytocin release (let-down or milk ejection reflex)
Adequate infant elimination patterns for age
Eagerness of infant to nurse
Maternal verbalization of satisfaction with the breastfeeding process

Breastfeeding, ineffective The state in which a mother, infant, and/or family experiences dissatisfaction or difficulty with the breastfeeding process.

Related factors

Prematurity
Infant anomaly
Maternal breast anomaly
Previous breast surgery
Previous history of breastfeeding failure
Infant receiving supplemental feedings with artificial nipple
Poor infant sucking reflex
Nonsupportive partner/family
Knowledge deficit
Interruption in breastfeeding

Defining characteristics

Unsatisfactory breastfeeding process
Actual or perceived inadequate milk supply
Infant's inability to attach on to maternal nipple correctly
No observable signs of oxytocin release
Observable signs of inadequate infant intake
Nonsustained suckling at breast
Suckling at only one breast per feeding
Nursing less than 7 times in 24 hours

Persistence of sore nipples beyond first week of infant's life

Maternal reluctance to put infant to breast as necessary

Infant exhibiting fussiness and crying within first hour after breastfeeding; unresponsive to other comfort measures

Infant arching and crying at breast; resisting latching on

Breastfeeding, interrupted
A break in the continuity of the breastfeeding process as a result of inability or inadvisability to put baby to breast for feeding.

Related factors
Maternal or infant illness

Prematurity

Maternal employment

Contraindications to breastfeeding (e.g., drugs, true breast-milk jaundice)

Need to abruptly wean infant

Defining Characteristics
Major
Infant does not receive nourishment at the breast for some or all of feedings

Minor
Maternal desire to maintain lactation and provide (or eventually provide) her breastmilk for her infant's nutritional needs

Separation of mother and infant

Lack of knowledge about expression and storage of breastmilk

Breathing pattern, ineffective
The state in which an individual's inhalation and/or exhalation pattern does not enable adequate ventilation.

Related factors
Neuromuscular impairment

Pain

Musculoskeletal impairment

Perception or cognitive impairment

Anxiety

Decreased energy and fatigue

Inflammatory process

Decreased lung expansion

Tracheobronchial obstruction

Defining characteristics
Dyspnea

Shortness of breath
Tachypnea
Fremitus
Abnormal arterial blood gas levels
Cyanosis
Cough
Nasal flaring
Respiratory depth changes
Assumption of three-point position
Pursed-lip breathing and prolonged expiratory phase
Increased anteroposterior diameter
Use of accessory muscles
Altered chest excursion

Cardiac output, decreased   The state in which the blood pumped by an individual's heart is sufficiently reduced to the extent that it is inadequate to meet the needs of the body's tissues.

Related factors
Mechanical
   Alteration in preload
   Alteration in afterload
   Alteration in inotropic changes in heart
Electrical
   Alteration in rate
   Alteration in rhythm
   Alteration in conduction
Structural

Defining characteristics
Variations in hemodynamic readings
Arrhythmias; ECG changes
Fatigue
Jugular vein distention
Cyanosis; pallor of skin and mucous membranes
Oliguria, anuria
Decreased peripheral pulses
Cold, clammy skin
Rales
Dyspnea

Caregiver role strain   A caregiver's felt difficulty in performing the family caregiver role.

Related factors
Pathophysiological/physiological
Severity of illness of the care receiver

Addiction or codependency

Premature birth/congenital defect

Discharge of family member with significant home health-care needs

Caregiver health impairment

Unpredictable illness course or instability in the care receiver's health

Gender of caregiver (female)

Developmental
Developmental inability to fulfill caregiver role (e.g., a young adult needing to provide care for a middle-aged parent)

Developmental delay or retardation of the care receiver or caregiver

Psychosocial
Psychological or cognitive problems in care receiver

Marginal family adaptation or dysfunction before caregiving became necessary

Marginal coping patterns of caregiver

History of poor relationship with care receiver

Spousal relationship to care receiver

Care receiver exhibits deviant, bizarre behavior

Situational
Presence of abuse or violence

Presence of situational stressors that normally affect families, such as significant loss, disaster or crisis, poverty or economic vulnerability, major life events (e.g., birth, hospitalization, leaving home, returning home, marriage, divorce, employment, retirement, and death)

Duration of caregiving required

Inadequate physical environment for providing care (e.g., housing, transportation, community services, equipment)

Isolation

Lack of respite and recreation

Inexperience with caregiving

Competing role commitments

Complexity/number of caregiving tasks

Defining Characteristics
Not having enough resources to provide the care needed

Finding it hard to do specific caregiving activities

Worry about such things as the care receiver's health and emotional state, having to put the care receiver in an institution, and who will care for the care receiver if something should happen to the caregiver

Feeling that caregiving interferes with other important roles in caregiver's life

Feeling loss because the care receiver is like a different person as compared with before caregiving began or, in the case of a child, that the care receiver was never the child the caregiver expected

Family conflict around issues of providing care

Stress or nervousness in the relationship with the care receiver

Depression

Caregiver role strain, high risk for   Vulnerability for feeling difficulty in performing the family caregiver role.

Risk factors
Pathophysiological
Severity of illness of the care receiver

Addiction or codependency

Premature birth/congenital defect

Discharge of family member with significant home health-care needs

Caregiver health impairment

Unpredictable illness course or instability in the care receiver's health

Gender of caregiver (female)

Psychological or cognitive problems in care receiver

Developmental
Developmental inability to fulfill caregiver role (e.g., a young adult needing to provide care for middle-aged parent)

Developmental delay or retardation of the care receiver or caregiver

Psychological
Marginal family adaptation or dysfunction before caregiving became necessary

Marginal coping patterns of caregiver

History of poor relationship with care receiver

Spousal relationship to care receiver

Care receiver exhibits deviant, bizarre behavior

Situational
Presence of abuse or violence

Presence of situational stressors that normally affect families, such as significant loss, disaster or crisis, poverty or economic vulnerability, major life events (e.g., birth, hospitalization, leaving home, returning home, marriage, divorce, employment, retirement, and death)

Duration of caregiving required

Inadequate physical environment for providing care (e.g., housing, transportation, community services, equipment)

Isolation

Lack of respite and recreation

Inexperience with caregiving

Competing role commitments

Complexity/number of caregiving tasks

Communication, impaired verbal   The state in which an individual experiences a decreased or absent ability to use or understand language in human interaction.

Related factors

Decrease in circulation to brain

Physical barrier, brain tumor, tracheostomy, intubation

Anatomic deficit, cleft palate

Psychological barriers, psychosis, lack of stimuli

Cultural difference

Developmental or age-related

Defining characteristics

Inability to speak dominant language

Refusal or inability to speak

Stuttering; slurring

Impaired articulation

Dyspnea

Disorientation

Inability to modulate speech

Inability to find words

Inability to name words

Inability to identify objects

Loose association of ideas

Flight of ideas

Incessant verbalization

Difficulty with phonation

Inability to speak in sentences

Constipation   The state in which an individual experiences a change in normal bowel habits characterized by a decrease in frequency and/or passage of hard, dry stools.

Related factors
Less than adequate intake
Less than adequate dietary intake and bulk
Less than adequate physical activity or immobility
Personal habits
Medications
Chronic use of medication and enemas
Gastrointestinal obstructive lesions
Neuromuscular impairment
Musculoskeletal impairment
Pain on defecation
Diagnostic procedures
Lack of privacy
Weak abdominal musculature
Pregnancy
Emotional status

Defining characteristics
Frequency less than usual pattern
Hard-formed stool
Palpable mass
Reported feeling of rectal fullness
Straining at stool
Decreased bowel sounds
Reported feeling of abdominal or rectal fullness or
   pressure
Less than usual amount of stool
Nausea

Other possible defining characteristics
Abdominal pain
Back pain
Headache
Interference with daily living
Use of laxatives
Decreased appetite
Appetite impairment

Constipation, colonic   The state in which an individual's
pattern of elimination is characterized by hard, dry stool that
results from a delay in passage of food residue.

Related factors
Less than adequate fluid intake
Less than adequate dietary intake
Less than adequate fiber intake

Less than adequate physical activity
Immobility
Lack of privacy
Emotional disturbances
Chronic use of medication and enemas
Stress
Change in daily routine
Metabolic problems (e.g., hypothyroidism, hypocalcemia, hypokalemia)

Defining characteristics
Decreased frequency
Hard, dry stool
Straining at stool
Painful defecation
Abdominal distention
Palpable mass
Rectal pressure
Headache, appetite impairment
Abdominal pain

Constipation, perceived   The state in which an individual makes a self-diagnosis of constipation and ensures a daily bowel movement through use of laxatives, enemas, and suppositories.

Related factors
Cultural/family health beliefs
Faulty appraisal
Impaired thought processes

Defining characteristics
Expectation of a daily bowel movement with resulting overuse of laxatives, enemas, and suppositories
Expected passage of stool at same time every day

Coping, defensive   The state in which an individual experiences falsely positive self-evaluation based on a self-protective pattern that defends against underlying perceived threats to positive self-regard.

Related factors
To be developed

Defining characteristics
Denial (of obvious problems/weaknesses)
Projection (of blame/responsibility)
Rationalization of failures
Defensiveness (hypersensitivity to criticism)

Grandiosity
Superior attitude toward others
Difficulty establishing/maintaining relationships
Hostile laughter or ridicule of others
Difficulty in reality testing of perceptions
Lack of follow-through or participation in treatment or therapy

Coping, family: potential for growth   Effective managing of adaptive tasks by family member involved with the patient's health challenge, who now is exhibiting desire and readiness for enhanced health and growth in regard to self and in relation to the patient.

Related factors

Family members attempt to describe growth impact of crisis on their own values, priorities, goals, or relationships.

Family member is moving in direction of health-promoting and enriching life-style that supports and monitors maturational processes, audits and negotiates treatment programs, and generally chooses experiences that optimize wellness.

Individual expresses interest in making contact on a one-to-one basis or on a mutual-aid group basis with another person who has experienced a similar situation.

Coping, ineffective family: compromised   Insufficient, ineffective, or compromised support, comfort, assistance, or encouragement—usually by a supportive primary person (family member or close friend); patient may need it to manage or master adaptive tasks related to his/her health challenge.

Related factors

Inadequate or incorrect information or understanding by a primary person

Temporary preoccupation by a significant person who is trying to manage emotional conflicts and personal suffering and is unable to perceive or act effectively in regard to patient's needs

Temporary family disorganization and role changes

Other situational or developmental crises or situations the significant person may be facing

Patient's providing little support for the primary person

Prolonged disease or disability progression that exhausts supportive capacity of significant people

Defining characteristics

Subjective

Patient expresses or confirms concern/complaint about significant other's response to patient's health problem

Significant person describes preoccupation with personal reactions (e.g., fear, anticipatory grief, guilt, anxiety) regarding patient's illness or disability or to other situational or developmental crises

Significant person describes or confirms an inadequate understanding or knowledge base that interferes with effective assistive or supportive behaviors

Objective

Significant person attempts assistive or supportive behaviors with less than satisfactory results

Significant person withdraws or enters into limited or temporary personal communication with patient at time of need

Significant person displays protective behavior disproportionate (too little or too much) to patient's abilities or need for autonomy

Coping, ineffective family: disabling
Behavior of significant person (family member or other primary person) that disables his/her own capacities and the patient's capacities to effectively address tasks essential to either person's adaptation to the health challenge.

Related factors

Significant person with chronically unexpressed feelings of guilt, anxiety, hostility, despair, etc.

Dissonant discrepancy of coping styles being used to deal with adaptive tasks by the significant person and patient or among significant people

Highly ambivalent family relationships

Arbitrary handling of family's resistance to treatment that tends to solidify defensiveness because it fails to deal adequately with underlying anxiety

Defining characteristics

Neglectful care of patient in regard to basic human needs and/or illness treatment

Distortion of reality about patient's health problem, including extreme denial about its existence or severity

Intolerance

Rejection

Abandonment
Desertion
Carrying on usual routines; disregarding patient's needs
Psychosomatic tendency
Taking on illness signs of patient
Decisions and actions by family that are detrimental to economic or social well-being
Agitation, depression, aggression, hostility
Impaired restructuring of a meaningful life for self; impaired individualization; prolonged overconcern for patient
Neglectful relationships with other family members
Patient's development of helpless, inactive dependence

Coping, ineffective individual Impairment of adaptive behaviors and problem-solving abilities of a person in meeting life's demands and roles.

Related factors
Situational crises
Maturational crises
Personal vulnerability
Multiple life changes
No vacations
Inadequate relaxation
Inadequate support systems
Little or no exercise
Poor nutrition
Unmet expectations
Work overload
Too many deadlines
Unrealistic perceptions
Inadequate coping method

Defining characteristics
Verbalization of inability to cope or inability to ask for help
Inability to meet role expectations
Inability to meet basic needs
Inability to problem solve
Alteration in societal participation
Destructive behavior toward self or others
Inappropriate use of defense mechanisms
Change in usual communication patterns
Verbal manipulation
High illness rate
High rate of accidents

Overeating
Lack of appetite
Excessive smoking
Excessive drinking
Overuse of prescribed tranquilizers
Alcohol proneness
High blood pressure
Chronic fatigue
Insomnia
Muscular tension
Ulcers
Frequent headaches
Frequent neckaches
Irritable bowel
Chronic worry
General irritability
Poor self-esteem
Chronic anxiety
Emotional tension
Chronic depression

Decisional conflict (specify)

A state of uncertainty about the course of action to be taken when choice among competing actions involves risk, loss, or challenge to personal life values. (Specify focus of conflict; e.g., choices regarding health, family relationships, career, finances, or other life events.)

Related factors

Unclear personal values/beliefs
Perceived threat to value system
Lack of experience or interference with decision making
Lack of relevant information
Support system deficit

Defining characteristics

Verbalized feeling of distress related to uncertainty about choices
Verbalization of undesired consequences of alternative actions being considered
Vacillation between alternative choices
Delayed decision making
Self-focusing
Physical signs of distress or tension (increased heart rate, increased muscle tension, restlessness, etc.)

Questioning personal values and beliefs while attempting to make a decision

Denial, ineffective A conscious or unconscious attempt to disavow the knowledge or meaning of an event to reduce anxiety/fear to the detriment of health.

Related factors
To be developed
Defining characteristics
Delay in seeking or refusal of medical attention to the detriment of health

Does not perceive personal relevance of symptoms or danger

Use of home remedies (self-treatment) to relieve symptoms

Does not admit fear of death or invalidism

Minimization of symptoms

Displacing source of symptoms to other organs

Inability to admit impact of disease on life pattern

Presence of dismissive gestures or comments when speaking of distressing events

Displacing fear of impact of condition

Inappropriate affect

Diarrhea The state in which an individual experiences a change in normal bowel habits characterized by the frequent passage of loose, fluid, unformed stools.

Related factors
Stress and anxiety

Dietary intake

Medications

Inflammation, irritation, or malabsorption of bowel

Toxins

Contaminants

Radiation
Defining characteristics
Abdominal pain

Cramping

Increased frequency of bowel movements

Increased frequency of bowel sounds

Loose, liquid stools

Urgency

Changes in color

Disuse syndrome, high risk for
The state in which an individual is at risk for deterioration of body systems as the result of prescribed or unavoidable inactivity.

Risk factors
Paralysis
Mechanical immobilization
Prescribed immobilization
Severe pain
Altered level of consciousness

Diversional activity deficit
The state in which an individual experiences a decreased stimulation from or interest or engagement in recreational or leisure activities.

Related factors
Environmental lack of diversional activity
Long-term hospitalization
Frequent, lengthy treatments
Defining characteristics
Boredom
Desire for something to do, to read, etc.
Usual hobbies cannot be undertaken in hospital

Dysreflexia
The state in which an individual with a spinal cord injury at T7 or above experiences or is at risk of experiencing a life-threatening uninhibited sympathetic response of the nervous system attributable to a noxious stimulus.

Related factors
To be developed
Defining characteristics
Individual with spinal cord injury (T7 or above) with the following:
Paroxysmal hypertension (sudden periodic elevated blood pressure where systolic pressure is over 140 mm Hg and diastolic pressure is above 90 mm Hg)
Bradycardia or tachycardia (pulse rate of less than 60 or over 100 beats per minute)
Diaphoresis (above injury)
Red splotches on skin (above injury)
Pallor (below injury)
Headache (diffuse pain in different portions of head and not confined to any nerve distribution area)
Chilling (shivering accompanied by sensation of coldness or pallor of skin)

Conjunctival congestion (excessive amount of blood/tissue fluid in conjunctivae)

Horner's syndrome (contraction of pupil, partial ptosis of eyelid, enophthalmos, and sometimes loss of sweating over affected side of face due to paralysis of cervical sympathetic nerve trunk)

Paresthesia (abnormal sensation, such as numbness, prickling, or tingling; increased sensitivity)

Pilomotor reflex (gooseflesh formation when skin is cooled)

Blurred vision

Chest pain

Metallic taste in mouth

Nasal congestion

Family processes, altered   The state in which a family that normally functions effectively experiences a dysfunction.

Related factors
Situational transition and/or crises

Developmental transition and/or crises

Defining characteristics*
Family system unable to meet physical needs of its members

Family system unable to meet emotional needs of its members

Family system unable to meet spiritual needs of its members

Parents do not demonstrate respect for each other's views on child-rearing practices

Inability to express or accept wide range of feelings

Inability to express or accept feelings of members

Family unable to meet security needs of its members

Inability of family members to relate to each other for mutual growth and maturation

Family uninvolved in community activities

Inability to accept or receive help appropriately

Rigidity in function and roles

Family does not demonstrate respect for individuality and autonomy of its members

Family unable to adapt to change or to deal with traumatic experience constructively

Family fails to accomplish current or past developmental task

Ineffective family decision-making process

Failure to send and receive clear messages

---

*The first 13 defining characteristics are specifically from Otto H: Criteria for assessing family strengths, *Fam Process* 2:329-338, Sept 1963.

Inappropriate boundary maintenance
Inappropriate or poorly communicated family rules, rituals,
   symbols
Unexamined family myths
Inappropriate level and direction of energy

Fatigue
An overwhelming sense of exhaustion and decreased capacity for physical and mental work regardless of adequate sleep.

Related factors
Overwhelming psychological or emotional demands
Increased energy requirements to perform activities of daily
   living
Excessive social/role demands
States of discomfort
Decreased metabolic energy production
Altered body chemistry (e.g., medications, drug withdrawal)

Defining characteristics
Verbalization of fatigue/lack of energy
Inability to maintain usual routines
Perceived need for additional energy to accomplish routine
   tasks
Increase in physical complaints
Emotional lability or irritability
Impaired ability to concentrate
Decreased performance
Lethargy or listlessness
Disinterest in surroundings/introspection
Decreased libido
Accident proneness

Fear
Feeling of dread related to an identifiable source that the person validates.

Related factors
Natural or innate origins—sudden noise, loss of physical
   support, height, pain
Learned response—conditioning, modeling from or identi-
   fication with others
Separation from support system in a potentially threatening
   situation (hospitalization, treatments, etc.)
Knowledge deficit or unfamiliarity
Language barrier
Sensory impairment

Phobic stimulus or phobia
Environmental stimuli
Defining characteristics
Subjective
Increased tension
Apprehension
Impulsiveness
Decreased self-assurance
Afraid
Scared
Terrified
Panicked
Frightened
Jittery
Objective
Increased alertness
Concentration on source
Wide-eyed
Attack behavior
Focus on "it, out there"
Fight behavior—aggressive
Flight behavior—withdrawal
Sympathetic stimulation—cardiovascular excitation, superficial vasoconstriction, pupil dilation

Fluid volume deficit (1) The state in which an individual experiences vascular, cellular, or intracellular dehydration related to failure of regulatory mechanisms.

Related factor
Failure of regulatory mechanisms
Defining characteristics
Dilute urine
Increased urine output
Sudden weight loss
Other possible defining characteristics
Possible weight gain
Hypotension
Decreased venous filling
Increased pulse rate
Decreased skin turgor
Decreased pulse volume and pressure
Increased body temperature
Dry skin

Dry mucous membranes
Hemoconcentration
Weakness
Edema
Thirst

Fluid volume deficit (2) The state in which an individual experiences vascular, cellular, or intracellular dehydration related to active loss.

Related factor
Active loss
Defining characteristics
Decreased urine output
Concentrated urine
Output greater than intake
Sudden weight loss
Decreased venous filling
Hemoconcentration
Increased serum sodium levels
Other possible defining characteristics
Hypotension
Thirst
Increased pulse rate
Decreased skin turgor
Decreased pulse volume and pressure
Change in mental state
Increased body temperature
Dry skin
Dry mucous membranes
Weakness

Fluid volume deficit, high risk for The state in which an individual is at risk of experiencing vascular, cellular, or intracellular dehydration.

Risk factors
Extremes of age
Extremes of weight
Excessive losses through normal routes (e.g., diarrhea)
Loss of fluid through abnormal routes (e.g., indwelling tubes)
Deviations affecting access to, intake of, or absorption of fluids (e.g., physical immobility)
Factors influencing fluid needs (e.g., hypermetabolic states)
Knowledge deficiency related to fluid volume

Medications (e.g., diuretics)
Increased fluid output
Urinary frequency
Thirst
Altered intake

Fluid volume excess
The state in which an individual experiences increased fluid retention and edema.

Related factors
Compromised regulatory mechanism
Excessive fluid intake
Excessive sodium intake

Defining characteristics
Edema
Effusion
Anasarca
Weight gain
Shortness of breath, orthopnea
Intake greater than output
Third heart sound
Pulmonary congestion on x-ray film
Abnormal breath sounds: crackles (rales)
Change in respiratory pattern
Change in mental status
Decreased hemoglobin, hematocrit levels
Blood pressure changes
Central venous pressure changes
Pulmonary artery pressure changes
Jugular venous distention
Positive hepatojugular reflex
Oliguria
Specific gravity changes
Azoturia
Altered electrolytes
Restlessness and anxiety

Gas exchange, impaired
The state in which an individual experiences an imbalance between oxygen uptake and carbon dioxide elimination at the alveolar-capillary membrane gas exchange area.

Related factors
Altered oxygen supply
Alveolar-capillary membrane changes

Altered blood flow
Altered oxygen-carrying capacity of blood
Defining characteristics
Confusion
Somnolence
Restlessness
Irritability
Inability to move secretions
Hypercapnia
Hypoxia

Grieving, anticipatory   The state in which an individual grieves before an actual loss.

Related factors
Perceived potential loss of significant other
Perceived potential loss of physiopsychosocial well-being
Perceived potential loss of personal possessions
Defining characteristics
Potential loss of significant object
Expression of distress at potential loss
Denial of potential loss
Guilt
Anger
Sorrow
Choked feelings
Changes in eating habits
Alterations in sleep patterns
Alterations in activity level
Altered libido
Altered communication patterns

Grieving, dysfunctional   The state in which actual or perceived object loss (object loss is used in the broadest sense) exists. Objects include people, possessions, a job, status, home, ideals, parts and processes of the body, etc.

Related factors
Actual or perceived object loss
Thwarted grieving response to a loss
Absence of anticipatory grieving
Chronic fatal illness
Lack of resolution of previous grieving response
Loss of significant others

Loss of physiopsychosocial well-being
Loss of personal possessions
Defining characteristics
Verbal expression of distress at loss
Denial of loss
Expression of guilt
Expression of unresolved issues
Anger
Sadness
Crying
Difficulty in expressing loss
Alterations in
  Eating habits
  Sleep patterns
  Dream patterns
  Activity level
  Libido
Idealization of lost object
Reliving of past experiences
Interference with life functioning
Developmental regression
Labile effect
Alterations in concentration and/or pursuits of tasks

Growth and development, altered
The state in which an individual demonstrates deviations in norms from his/her age-group.

Related factors
Inadequate caretaking: indifference, inconsistent responsiveness, multiple caretakers
Separation from significant others
Environmental and stimulation deficiencies
Effects of physical disability
Prescribed dependence
Defining characteristics
Delay or difficulty in performing skills (motor, social, or expressive) typical of age-group
Altered physical growth
Inability to perform self-care or self-control activities appropriate for age
Flat affect
Listlessness, decreased responses

Health maintenance, altered Inability to identify, manage, and/or seek help to maintain health.

Related factors
Lack of or significant alteration in communication skills (written, verbal, and/or gestural)

Lack of ability to make deliberate and thoughtful judgments

Perceptual or cognitive impairment

Complete or partial lack of gross and/or fine motor skills

Ineffective individual coping; dysfunctional grieving

Lack of material resources

Unachieved developmental tasks

Ineffective family coping; disabling spiritual distress

Defining characteristics
Demonstrated lack of knowledge regarding basic health practices

Demonstrated lack of adaptive behaviors to internal or external environmental changes

Reported or observed inability to take responsibility for meeting basic health practices in any or all functional pattern areas

History of lack of health-seeking behavior

Expressed interest in improving health behaviors

Reported or observed lack of equipment, financial, and/or other resources

Reported or observed impairment of personal support system

Health-seeking behaviors (specify) The state in which a patient in stable health is actively seeking ways to alter personal health habits and/or the environment in order to move toward optimal health. (*Stable health status* is defined as age-appropriate illness prevention measures achieved; the patient reports good or excellent health, and signs and symptoms of disease, if present, are controlled.)

Related factors
To be developed

Defining characteristics
Expressed or observed desire to seek higher level of wellness

Stated or observed unfamiliarity with wellness community resources

Demonstrated or observed lack of knowledge in health promotion behaviors

Expressed or observed desire for increased control of health practice

Expression of concern about effects of current environmental conditions on health status

Home maintenance management, impaired   Inability to independently maintain a safe growth-promoting immediate environment.

Related factors
Disease or injury of individual or family member
Insufficient family organization or planning
Insufficient finances
Unfamiliarity with neighborhood resources
Impaired cognitive or emotional functioning
Lack of knowledge
Lack of role modeling
Inadequate support systems

Defining characteristics
Subjective
    Household members express difficulty in maintaining their home in a comfortable fashion
    Household requests assistance with home maintenance
    Household members describe outstanding debts or financial crises
Objective
    Disorderly surroundings
    Unwashed or unavailable cooking equipment, clothes, or linen
    Accumulation of dirt, food wastes, or hygienic wastes
    Offensive odors
    Inappropriate household temperature
    Overtaxed family members (e.g., exhausted, anxious family members)
    Lack of necessary equipment or aids
    Presence of vermin or rodents
    Repeated hygienic disorders, infestations, or infections

Hopelessness   The subjective state in which an individual sees limited or no alternatives or personal choices available and is unable to mobilize energy on own behalf.

Related factors
Prolonged activity restriction creating isolation

Failing or deteriorating physiological condition
Long-term stress
Abandonment
Loss of belief in transcendent values/God
Defining characteristics
Passivity, decreased verbalization
Decreased affect
Verbal cues (indicating despondency, "I can't," sighing)
Lack of initiative
Decreased response to stimuli
Turning away from speaker
Closing eyes
Shrugging in response to speaker
Decreased appetite; increased/decreased sleep
Lack of involvement in care; passively allowing care

Hyperthermia   The state in which an individual's body temperature is elevated above his/her normal range.

Related factors
Exposure to hot environment
Vigorous activity
Medications/anesthesia
Inappropriate clothing
Increased metabolic rate
Illness or trauma
Dehydration
Inability or decreased ability to perspire
Defining characteristics
Increase in body temperature above normal range
Flushed skin
Warm to touch
Increased respiratory rate
Tachycardia
Seizures/convulsions

Hypothermia   The state in which an individual's body temperature is reduced below his/her normal range but not below 35.6° C (rectal)/36.4° C (rectal, newborn).

Related factors
Exposure to cool or cold environment
Illness or trauma
Inability or decreased ability to shiver

Malnutrition
Inadequate clothing
Consumption of alcohol
Medications causing vasodilation
Evaporation from skin in cool environment
Decreased metabolic rate
Inactivity
Aging

Defining characteristics
Shivering (mild)
Cool skin
Pallor (moderate)
Slow capillary refill
Tachycardia
Cyanotic nail beds
Hypertension
Piloerection

Incontinence, bowel See Bowel incontinence.

Incontinence, functional The state in which an individual experiences an involuntary, unpredictable passage of urine.

Related factors
Altered environment
Sensory, cognitive, or mobility deficits

Defining characteristics
Urge to void or bladder contractions sufficiently strong to result in loss of urine before reaching an appropriate receptacle

Incontinence, reflex The state in which an individual experiences an involuntary loss of urine occurring at somewhat predictable intervals when a specific bladder volume is reached.

Related factor
Neurological impairment (e.g., spinal cord lesion that interferes with conduction of cerebral messages above level of reflex arc)

Defining characteristics
No awareness of bladder filling
No urge to void or feelings of bladder fullness
Uninhibited bladder contraction/spasm at regular intervals

Incontinence, stress   The state in which an individual experiences a loss of urine of less than 50 ml occurring with increased abdominal pressure.

Related factors

Degenerative changes in pelvic muscles and structural supports associated with increased age

High intraabdominal pressure (e.g., obesity, gravid uterus)

Incompetent bladder outlet

Overdistention between voidings

Weak pelvic muscles and structural supports

Defining characteristics

Reported or observed dribbling with increased abdominal pressure

Urinary urgency

Urinary frequency (more often than every 2 hours)

Incontinence, total   The state in which an individual experiences a continuous and unpredictable loss of urine.

Related factors

Neuropathy preventing transmission of reflex indicating bladder fullness

Neurological dysfunction causing triggering of micturition at unpredictable times

Independent contraction of detrusor reflex due to surgery

Trauma or disease affecting spinal cord nerves

Anatomic (fistula)

Defining characteristics

Constant flow of urine occurring at unpredictable times without distention or uninhibited bladder contractions/spasms

Unsuccessful incontinence refractory to treatments

Nocturia

Lack of perineal or bladder-filling awareness

Unawareness of incontinence

Incontinence, urge   The state in which an individual experiences involuntary passage of urine occurring soon after a strong sense of urgency to void.

Related factors

Decreased bladder capacity (e.g., history of PID, abdominal surgeries, indwelling urinary catheter)

Irritation of bladder stretch receptors, causing spasm (e.g., bladder infection)

Alcohol
Caffeine
Increased fluids
Increased urine concentration
Overdistention of bladder

Defining characteristics
Urinary urgency
Frequency (voiding more often than every 2 hours)
Bladder contracture/spasm
Nocturia (more than 2 times per night)
Voiding in small (less than 100 ml) or in large amounts (more than 550 ml)
Inability to reach toilet in time

Infant feeding pattern, ineffective
A state in which an infant demonstrates an impaired ability to suck or coordinate the suck-swallow response.

Related factors
Prematurity
Neurological impairment/delay
Oral hypersensitivity
Prolonged NPO status
Anatomic abnormality

Defining characteristics
Inability to initiate or sustain an effective suck
Inability to coordinate sucking, swallowing, and breathing

Infection, high risk for
The state in which an individual is at increased risk for being invaded by pathogenic organisms.

Risk factors
Inadequate primary defenses (broken skin, traumatized tissue, decrease in ciliary action, stasis of body fluids, change in pH secretions, altered peristalsis)
Inadequate secondary defenses (e.g., decreased hemoglobin level, leukopenia, suppressed inflammatory response, immunosuppression)
Inadequate acquired immunity
Tissue destruction and increased environmental exposure
Chronic disease
Invasive procedures
Malnutrition

Pharmaceutical agents and trauma

Rupture of amniotic membranes

Insufficient knowledge to avoid exposure to pathogens

Injury, high risk for The state in which an individual is at risk of injury as a result of environmental conditions interacting with the individual's adaptive and defensive resources. See also Poisoning, high risk for; Suffocation, high risk for; Trauma, high risk for.

Risk factors

Interactive conditions between individual and environment that impose a risk to defensive and adaptive resources of individual

Internal

Biochemical

Regulatory function

Sensory dysfunction

Integrative dysfunction

Effector dysfunction

Tissue hypoxia

Malnutrition

Immune-autoimmune

Abnormal blood profile

Leukocytosis or leukopenia

Altered clotting factors

Thrombocytopenia

Sickle cell

Thalassemia

Decreased hemoglobin level

Physical

Broken skin

Altered mobility

Developmental

Age

Physiological

Psychosocial

Psychological

Affective

Orientation

External

Biological

Immunization level of community

Microorganism

Chemical
  Pollutants
  Poisons
  Drugs
    Pharmaceutical agents
    Alcohol
    Caffeine
    Nicotine
  Preservatives
  Cosmetics and dyes
  Nutrients (vitamins, food types)
Physical
  Design, structure, and arrangement of community, building, and/or equipment
  Mode of transport/transportation
  Nosocomial agents
People-provider
  Nosocomial agents
  Staffing patterns
  Cognitive, affective, and psychomotor factors

Knowledge deficit (specify)   The state in which specific information is lacking.

Related factors
Lack of exposure
Lack of recall
Information misinterpretation
Cognitive limitation
Lack of interest in learning
Unfamiliarity with information resources
Patient's request for no information

Defining characteristics
Verbalization of the problem
Inaccurate follow-through of instruction
Inadequate performance of test
Inappropriate or exaggerated behaviors (e.g., hysterical, hostile, agitated, apathetic)
Statement of misconception
Request for information

Management of therapeutic regimen (individuals), ineffective   A pattern of regulating and integrating into daily living a program for treatment of illness and the sequelae of illness that is unsatisfactory for meeting specific health goals.

Related factors

Complexity of health care system
Complexity of therapeutic regimen
Decisional conflicts
Economic difficulties
Excessive demands made on individual or family
Family conflict
Family patterns of health care
Inadequate number and types of cues to action
Knowledge deficits
Mistrust of regimen and/or health care personnel
Perceived seriousness
Perceived susceptibility
Perceived barriers
Perceived benefits
Powerlessness
Social support deficits

Defining characteristics

Major

Choices of daily living ineffective for meeting the goals of a
treatment or prevention program

Minor

Acceleration (expected or unexpected) of illness symptoms
Verbalized desire to manage the treatment of illness and prevention of sequelae
Verbalized difficulty with regulation/integration of one or
more prescribed regimens for treatment of illness and its
effects or prevention of complications
Verbalization that intimated that patient would not attempt to
include treatment regimens in daily routines
Verbalization that intimated that patient would not attempt to
reduce risk factors for progression of illness and sequelae

Mobility, impaired physical   The state in which an in-
dividual experiences a limitation of ability for independent
physical movement.

Related factors

Intolerance to activity; decreased strength and endurance
Pain and discomfort
Perceptual or cognitive impairment
Neuromuscular impairment
Musculoskeletal impairment
Depression; severe anxiety

Defining characteristics

Inability to purposefully move within physical environment, including bed mobility, transfer, and ambulation

Reluctance to attempt movement

Limited range of motion

Decreased muscle strength, control, and/or mass

Imposed restrictions of movement, including mechanical; medical protocol

Impaired coordination

Noncompliance (specify) A person's informed decision not to adhere to a therapeutic recommendation.

Related factors

Patient's value system

Health beliefs

Cultural influences

Spiritual values

Client and provider relationships

Defining characteristics

Behavior indicative of failure to adhere by direct observation or statements by patient or significant others

Objective tests (physiological measures, detection of markers)

Evidence of development of complications

Evidence of exacerbation of symptoms

Failure to keep appointments

Failure to progress

Inability to set or attain mutual goals

Nutrition, altered: less than body requirements

The state in which an individual experiences an intake of nutrients insufficient to meet metabolic needs.

Related factor

Inability to ingest or digest food or absorb nutrients because of biological, psychological, or economic factors

Defining characteristics

Loss of weight with adequate food intake

Body weight 20% or more under ideal for height and frame

Reported inadequate food intake less than Recommended Daily Allowance

Weakness of muscles required for swallowing or mastication

Reported or evidence of lack of food

Lack of interest in food

Perceived inability to ingest food

Aversion to eating
Reported altered taste sensation
Satiety immediately after ingesting food
Abdominal pain with or without pathological conditions
Sore, inflamed buccal cavity

Nutrition, altered: more than body requirements

The state in which an individual is experiencing an intake of nutrients that exceeds metabolic needs.

Related factor

Excessive intake in relationship to metabolic need

Defining characteristics

Weight 10%-20% over ideal for height and frame

Triceps skinfold greater than 15 mm in men and 25 mm in women

Sedentary activity level

Reported or observed dysfunctional eating patterns

Pairing food with other activities

Concentrating food intake at end of day

Eating in response to external cues (e.g., time of day, social situation)

Eating in response to internal cues other than hunger (e.g., anxiety)

Nutrition, altered: high risk for more than body requirements The state in which an individual is at risk of experiencing an intake of nutrients that exceeds metabolic needs.

Risk factors

Hereditary predisposition

Excessive energy intake during late gestational life, early infancy, and adolescence

Frequent, closely spaced pregnancies

Dysfunctional psychological conditioning in relationship to food

Membership in lower socioeconomic group

Reported or observed obesity in one or both parents

Rapid transition across growth percentiles in infants or children

Reported use of solid food as major food source before 5 months of age

Observed use of food as reward or comfort measure

Reported or observed higher baseline weight at beginning of each pregnancy

Dysfunctional eating patterns

Pairing food with other activities

Concentrating food intake at end of day

Eating in response to external cues (e.g., time of day or social situation)

Eating in response to internal cues other than hunger (e.g., anxiety)

Oral mucous membrane, altered
The state in which an individual experiences disruptions in the tissue layers of the oral cavity.

Related factors
Pathological conditions—oral cavity (radiation to head and/or neck)

Dehydration

Trauma

Chemical (e.g., acidic foods, drugs, noxious agents, alcohol)

Mechanical (e.g., ill-fitting dentures; braces; tubes—endotracheal, nasogastric; surgery in oral cavity)

NPO instructions for more than 24 hours

Ineffective oral hygiene

Mouth breathing

Malnutrition

Infection

Lack of or decreased salivation

Medication

Defining characteristics
Coated tongue

Xerostomia (dry mouth)

Stomatitis

Oral lesions or ulcers

Lack of or decreased salivation

Leukoplakia

Edema

Hyperemia

Oral plaque

Oral pain or discomfort

Desquamation

Vesicles

Hemorrhagic gingivitis

Carious teeth

Halitosis

Pain The state in which an individual experiences and reports the presence of severe discomfort or an uncomfortable sensation.

Related factors

Injuring agents

Biological

Chemical

Physical

Psychological

Defining characteristics

Subjective

Communication (verbal or coded) of pain descriptors

Objective

Guarding behavior; protective

Self-focusing

Narrowed focus (altered time perception, withdrawal from social contact, impaired thought process)

Distraction behavior (moaning, crying, pacing, seeking other people and/or activities, restlessness)

Facial mask of pain (eyes lack luster, "beaten look," fixed or scattered movement, grimace)

Alteration in muscle tone (may span from listless to rigid)

Autonomic responses not seen in chronic, stable pain (diaphoresis, blood pressure and pulse rate change, pupillary dilation, increased or decreased respiratory rate)

Pain, chronic The state in which an individual experiences pain that continues for more than 6 months.

Related factor

Chronic physical/psychosocial disability

Defining characteristics

Verbal report or observed evidence of pain experienced for more than 6 months

Fear of reinjury

Physical and social withdrawal

Altered ability to continue previous activities

Anorexia

Weight changes

Changes in sleep patterns

Facial masks
Guarded movement

Parental role conflict The state in which a parent experiences role confusion and conflict in response to a crisis.

Related factors
Separation from child due to chronic illness
Intimidation with invasive or restrictive modalities (e.g., isolation, intubation)
Specialized care centers, policies
Home care of a child with special needs (e.g., apnea monitoring, postural drainage, hyperalimentation)
Change in marital status
Interruptions of family life due to home health-care regimen (treatments, caregivers, lack of respite)

Defining characteristics
Parent(s) expresses concerns/feelings of inadequacy to provide for child's physical and emotional needs during hospitalization or in home
Demonstrated disruption in caretaking routines
Parent(s) expresses concerns about changes in parental role, family functioning, family communication, and/or family health
Expresses concern about perceived loss of control over decisions relating to child
Reluctant to participate in normal caretaking activities even with encouragement and support
Verbalizes/demonstrates feelings of guilt, anger, fear, anxiety, and/or frustrations about effect of child's illness on family process

Parenting, altered
Parenting, altered, high risk for The state in which the ability of nurturing figure(s) to create an environment that promotes the optimal growth and development of another human being is altered or at risk.

Related/risk factors
Lack of available role model
Ineffective role model
Physical and psychosocial abuse of nurturing figure
Lack of support between or from significant other(s)
Unmet social and emotional maturation needs of parenting figures

Interruption in bonding process (i.e., maternal, paternal, other)

Perceived threat to own survival: physical and emotional

Mental and/or physical illness

Presence of stress: financial or legal problems, recent crisis, cultural move

Lack of knowledge

Limited cognitive functioning

Lack of role identity

Lack of appropriate response of child to relationship

Multiple pregnancies

Unrealistic expectation of self, infant, partner

Defining characteristics

Actual and potential

Lack of parental attachment behaviors

Inappropriate visual, tactile, auditory stimulation

Negative identification of characteristics of infant/child

Negative attachment of meanings to characteristics of infant/child

Constant verbalization of disappointment in gender or physical characteristics of infant/child

Verbalization of resentment toward infant/child

Verbalization of role inadequacy

Inattention to needs of infant/child

Verbal disgust at body functions of infant/child

Noncompliance with health appointments for self and/or infant/child

Inappropriate caretaking behaviors (toilet training, sleep and rest, feeding)

Inappropriate or inconsistent discipline practices

Frequent accidents

Frequent illness

Growth and development lag in child

History of child abuse or abandonment by primary caretaker

Verbalizes desire to have child call parent by first name despite traditional cultural tendencies

Child receives care from multiple caretakers without consideration for needs of child

Compulsive seeking of role approval from others

Actual

Abandonment

Runaway

Verbalization of inability to control child
Evidence of physical and psychological trauma

Peripheral neurovascular dysfunction, high risk for
A state in which an individual is at risk of experiencing a disruption in circulation, sensation, or motion of an extremity.

Risk factors
Fractures
Mechanical compression (e.g., tourniquet, cast, brace, dressing, or restraint)
Orthopedic surgery
Trauma
Immobilization
Burns
Vascular obstruction

Personal identity disturbance
Inability to distinguish between self and nonself.

Related factors
To be developed
Defining characteristics
To be developed

Poisoning, high risk for
Accentuated risk of accidental exposure to or ingestion of drugs or dangerous products in doses sufficient to cause poisoning.

Risk factors
Internal (individual) factors
Reduced vision
Verbalization of occupational setting without adequate safeguards
Lack of safety or drug education
Lack of proper precaution
Cognitive or emotional difficulties
Insufficient finances
External (environmental) factors
Large supplies of drugs in house
Medicines stored in unlocked cabinets accessible to children or confused persons
Dangerous products placed or stored within reach of children or confused persons
Availability of illicit drugs potentially contaminated by poisonous additives

Flaking, peeling paint or plaster in presence of young children

Chemical contamination of food and water

Unprotected contact with heavy metals or chemicals

Paint, lacquer, etc., in poorly ventilated areas or without effective protection

Presence of poisonous vegetation

Presence of atmospheric pollutants

Post-trauma response
The state in which an individual experiences a sustained painful response to (an) overwhelming traumatic event(s).

Related factors
Disaster

War

Epidemic

Rape

Assault

Torture

Catastrophic illness

Accident

Defining characteristics
Reexperience of traumatic event, which may be identified in cognitive, affective, and/or sensory motor activities (flashbacks, intrusive thoughts, repetitive dreams or nightmares, excessive verbalization of traumatic event, verbalization of survival guilt or guilt about behavior required for survival)

Psychic/emotional numbness (impaired interpretation of reality, confusion, dissociation or amnesia, vagueness about traumatic event, constricted affect)

Altered life-style (self-destructiveness, such as substance abuse, suicide attempt, or other acting-out behavior; difficulty with interpersonal relationships; development of phobia regarding trauma; poor impulse control/irritability; explosiveness)

Powerlessness
Perception that one's own action will not significantly affect an outcome; a perceived lack of control over a current situation or immediate happening.

Related factors
Health-care environment

Interpersonal interaction

Illness-related regimen

Life-style of helplessness

Defining characteristics

Severe

Verbal expressions of having no control or influence over situation

Verbal expressions of having no control or influence over outcome

Verbal expressions of having no control over self-care

Depression over physical deterioration that occurs despite patient compliance with regimens

Apathy

Moderate

Nonparticipation in care or decision making when opportunities are provided

Expressions of dissatisfaction and frustration over inability to perform previous tasks and/or activities

Does not monitor progress

Expression of doubt regarding role performance

Reluctance to express true feelings, fearing alienation from caregivers

Inability to seek information regarding care

Dependence on others that may result in irritability, resentment, anger, and guilt

Does not defend self-care practices when challenged

Low

Passivity

Expressions of uncertainty about fluctuating energy levels

Protection, altered   The state in which an individual experiences a decrease in the ability to guard the self from internal or external threats, such as illness or injury.

Related factors

Extremes of age

Inadequate nutrition

Alcohol abuse

Abnormal blood profiles (leukopenia, thrombocytopenia, anemia, coagulation)

Drug therapies (antineoplastic, cortiocosteroid, immune, anticoagulant, thrombolytic)

Treatments (surgery, radiation)

Diseases such as cancer and immune disorders

Defining characteristics
Deficient immunity
Impaired healing
Altered clotting
Maladaptive stress response
Neurosensory alterations
Chilling
Perspiring
Dyspnea
Cough
Itching
Restlessness
Insomnia
Fatigue
Anorexia
Weakness
Immobility
Disorientation
Pressure sores

Rape-trauma syndrome   Forced, violent sexual penetration against the victim's will and consent. The trauma syndrome that develops from this attack or attempted attack includes an acute phase or disorganization of the victim's life-style and a long-term process of reorganization of life-style.

Related factors
Inadequate support systems
Spouse-family blaming
Fear of reprisal, pregnancy, going out alone
Anxiety about potential health problems (e.g., AIDS, venereal disease, herpes)

Defining characteristics
Acute phase
  Emotional reactions
    Anger
    Embarrassment
    Fear of physical violence and death
    Humiliation
    Revenge
    Self-blame
  Multiple physical symptoms
  Gastrointestinal irritability
  Genitourinary discomfort

Muscle tension

Sleep pattern disturbance

Long-term phase

Changes in life-style (changes in residence; dealing with repetitive nightmares and phobias; seeking family support; seeking social network support)

Rape-trauma syndrome: compound reaction

An acute stress reaction to a rape or attempted rape, experienced along with other major stressors, that can include reactivation of symptoms of a previous condition.*

Related factors

Drug or alcohol abuse

History of and/or current psychiatric illness

History of and/or current physical illness

Defining characteristics

All defining characteristics listed under Rape-Trauma Syndrome

Reactivated symptoms of such previous conditions (i.e., physical illness, psychiatric illness)

Reliance on alcohol and/or drugs

Rape-trauma syndrome: silent reaction

A complex stress reaction to a rape in which an individual is unable to describe or discuss the rape.*

Related factors

Fear of retaliation

Intense shame

Excessive denial

Lack of support

Defining characteristics

Abrupt changes in relationships with members of the opposite sex

Increase in nightmares

Increasing anxiety during interview (e.g., blocking of associations, long periods of silence, minor stuttering, physical distress)

Marked changes in sexual behavior

No verbalization of occurrence of the rape

Sudden onset of phobic reactions

*Definition developed by Kim, McFarland, and McLane.

Relocation stress syndrome
Physiological and/or psychosocial disturbances as a result of transfer from one environment to another.

Related factors
Past, concurrent, and recent losses
Losses involved with decision to move
Feeling of powerlessness
Lack of adequate support system
Little or no preparation for the impending move
Moderate to high degree of environmental change
History and types of previous transfers
Impaired psychosocial health status
Decreased physical health status

Defining characteristics
Major
Change in environment/location
Anxiety
Apprehension
Increased confusion (elderly population)
Depression
Loneliness
Minor
Verbalization of unwillingness to relocate
Sleep disturbance
Change in eating habits
Dependency
Gastrointestinal disturbances
Increased verbalization of needs
Insecurity
Lack of trust
Restlessness
Sad affect
Unfavorable comparison of post/pre-transfer staff
Verbalization of being concerned/upset about transfer
Vigilance
Weight change
Withdrawal

Role performance, altered
Disruption in the way one perceives one's role performance.

Related factors
To be developed

Defining characteristics
Change in self-perception of role
Denial of role
Change in others' perception of role
Conflict in roles
Change in physical capacity to resume role
Lack of knowledge of role
Change in usual patterns or responsibility

Self-care deficit, bathing/hygiene The state in which one experiences an impaired ability to perform or complete bathing/hygiene activities for oneself.

Related factors
To be developed
Defining characteristics
Inability to wash body or body parts
Inability to obtain or get to water source
Inability to regulate temperature or flow

Self-care deficit, dressing/grooming The state in which one experiences an impaired ability to perform or complete dressing and grooming activities for onself.

Related factors
To be developed
Defining characteristics
Impaired ability to put on or take off necessary items of clothing
Impaired ability to obtain or replace articles of clothing
Impaired ability to fasten clothing
Inability to maintain appearance at satisfactory level

Self-care deficit, feeding The state in which one experiences an impaired ability to perform or complete feeding activities for oneself.

Related factors
To be developed
Defining characteristic
Inability to bring food from receptacle to mouth

Self-care deficit, toileting The state in which one experiences an impaired ability to perform or complete toileting activities for oneself.

Related factors

Impaired transfer ability

Impaired mobility status

Intolerance to activity; decreased strength and endurance

Pain, discomfort

Perceptual or cognitive impairment

Neuromuscular impairment

Musculoskeletal impairment

Depression, severe anxiety

Defining characteristics

Inability to get to toilet or commode

Inability to sit on or rise from toilet or commode

Inability to manipulate clothing for toileting

Inability to carry out proper toilet hygiene

Inability to flush toilet or empty commode

Self-concept, disturbance in See Body Image Disturbance; Personal Identity Disturbance; Self-Esteem Disturbance.

Self-esteem disturbance Negative self-evaluation/feelings about self or self-capabilities, which may be directly or indirectly expressed.

Related factors

To be developed

Defining characteristics

Self-negating verbalization

Expressions of shame/guilt

Evaluation of self as unable to deal with events

Rationalization/rejection of positive feedback and exaggeration of negative feedback about self

Hesitancy to try new things/situations

Denial of problems obvious to others

Projection of blame/responsibility for problems

Rationalization of personal failures

Hypersensitivity to criticism

Grandiosity

Self-esteem, chronic low Long-standing negative self-evaluation/feelings about self or self-capabilities.

Related factors

To be developed

Defining characteristics
Self-negating verbalization

Expressions of shame/guilt

Evaluation of self as unable to deal with events

Rationalization/rejection of positive feedback and exaggeration of negative feedback about self

Hesitancy to try new things/situations

Frequent lack of success in work or other life events

Overly conforming; dependence on others' opinions

Lack of eye contact

Nonassertive/passive

Indecisive

Excessively seeks reassurance

Self-esteem, situational low
Negative self-evaluation/ feelings about self that develop in response to a loss or change in an individual who previously had a positive self-evaluation.

Related factors
To be developed

Defining characteristics
Episodic occurrence of negative self-appraisal in response to life events in a person with a previous positive self-evaluation

Verbalization of negative feelings about self (helplessness, uselessness)

Self-negating verbalizations

Expressions of shame/guilt

Evaluation of self as unable to handle situations/events

Difficulty making decisions

Self-mutilation, high risk for
A state in which an individual is at high risk to perform an act on the self to injure, not kill, that produces tissue damage and tension relief.

Risk factors
Groups at risk:

Clients with borderline personality disorder, especially females 16 to 25 years of age

Clients in psychotic state—frequently males in young adulthood

Emotionally disturbed and/or battered children

Mentally retarded and autistic children

Clients with a history of self-injury

History of physical, emotional, or sexual abuse

Inability to cope with increased psychological/physiological tension in a healthy manner

Feelings of depression, rejection, self-hatred, separation anxiety, guilt, and depersonalization

Fluctuating emotions

Command hallucinations

Need for sensory stimuli

Parental emotional deprivation

Dysfunctional family

Sensory/perceptual alterations (specify) (visual, auditory, kinesthetic, gustatory, tactile, olfactory)

The state in which an individual experiences a change in the amount or patterning of incoming stimuli accompanied by a diminished, exaggerated, distorted, or impaired response to such stimuli.

Related factors

Environmental factors

Therapeutically restricted environments (isolation, intensive care, bed rest, traction, confining illnesses, incubator)

Socially restricted environment (institutionalization, homebound, aging, chronic illness, dying, infant deprivation); stigmatized (mentally ill, mentally retarded, mentally handicapped); bereaved

Altered sensory reception, transmission, and/or integration

Neurological disease, trauma, or deficit

Altered status of sense organs

Inability to communicate, understand, speak, or respond

Sleep deprivation

Pain

Chemical alteration

Endogenous (electrolyte imbalance, elevated BUN level, elevated ammonia, hypoxia)

Exogenous (central nervous system stimulants or depressants, mind-altering drugs)

Psychological stress (narrowed perceptual fields caused by anxiety)

Defining characteristics

Disoriented in time, in place, or with persons

Altered abstraction

Altered conceptualization

Change in problem-solving abilities

Reported or measured change in sensory acuity
Change in behavior pattern
Anxiety
Apathy
Change in usual response to stimuli
Indication of body image alteration
Restlessness
Irritability
Altered communication patterns
Disorientation
Lack of concentration
Daydreaming
Hallucinations
Noncompliance
Fear
Depression
Rapid mood swings
Anger
Exaggerated emotional responses
Poor concentration
Disordered thought sequencing
Bizarre thinking
Visual and auditory distortions
Motor incoordination

Other possible defining characteristics

Complaints of fatigue
Alteration in posture
Change in muscular tension
Inappropriate responses
Hallucinations

Sexual dysfunction The state in which an individual experiences a change in sexual function that is viewed as unsatisfying, unrewarding, or inadequate.

Related factors

Biopsychosocial alteration of sexuality
Ineffectual or absent role models
Physical abuse
Psychosocial abuse (e.g., harmful relationships)
Vulnerability
Misinformation or lack of knowledge
Values conflict
Lack of privacy

Lack of significant other

Altered body structure or function: pregnancy, recent child-birth, drugs, surgery, anomalies, disease process, trauma, radiation

Defining characteristics

Verbalization of problem

Alterations in achieving perceived sex role

Actual or perceived limitation imposed by disease and/or therapy

Conflicts involving values

Alterations in achieving sexual satisfaction

Inability to achieve desired satisfaction

Seeking of confirmation of desirability

Alteration in relationship with significant other

Change in interest in self and others

Sexuality patterns, altered   The state in which an individual expresses concern regarding his/her sexuality.

Related factors

Knowledge/skill deficit about alternative responses to health-related transitions, altered body function or structure, illness, or medical treatment

Lack of privacy

Lack of significant other

Ineffective or absent role models

Conflicts with sexual orientation or variant preferences

Fear of pregnancy or of acquiring sexually transmitted disease

Impaired relationship with significant other

Defining characteristic

Reported difficulties, limitations, or changes in sexual behaviors or activities

Skin integrity, impaired   The state in which an individual's skin is adversely altered.

Related factors

External (environmental)

Hyperthermia or hypothermia

Chemical substance

Mechanical factors

Shearing forces

Pressure

Restraint

Radiation
Physical immobilization
Humidity
Internal (somatic)
Medication
Altered nutritional state: obesity, emaciation
Altered metabolic state
Altered circulation
Altered sensation
Altered pigmentation
Skeletal prominence
Developmental factors
Immunological deficit
Alterations in turgor (change in elasticity)
Excretions/secretions
Psychogenic
Edema

Defining characteristics
Disruption of skin surface
Destruction of skin layers
Invasion of body structures

Skin integrity, impaired, high risk for
The state in which an individual's skin is at risk of being adversely altered.

Risk factors
External (environmental)
Hypothermia or hyperthermia
Chemical substance
Mechanical factors
Shearing forces
Pressure
Restraint
Radiation
Physical immobilization
Excretions and secretions
Humidity
Internal (somatic)
Medication
Alterations in nutritional state (obesity, emaciation)
Altered metabolic state
Altered circulation
Altered sensation
Altered pigmentation

Skeletal prominence
Developmental factors
Alterations in skin turgor (change in elasticity)
Psychogenic
Immunological

Sleep pattern disturbance
Disruption of sleep time causes discomfort or interferes with desired life-style.

Related factors
Sensory alterations
  Internal factors
    Illness
    Psychological stress
  External factors
    Environmental changes
    Social cues

Defining characteristics
Verbal complaints of difficulty in falling asleep
Awakening earlier or later than desired
Interrupted sleep
Verbal complaints of not feeling well rested
Changes in behavior and performance
  Increasing irritability
  Restlessness
  Disorientation
  Lethargy
  Listlessness
Physical signs
  Mild, fleeting nystagmus
  Slight hand tremor
  Ptosis of eyelid
  Expressionless face
Thick speech with mispronunciation and incorrect words
Dark circles under eyes
Frequent yawning
Changes in posture
Not feeling well rested

Social interaction, impaired
The state in which an individual participates in an insufficient or excessive quantity or ineffective quality of social exchange.

Related factors
Knowledge/skill deficit about ways to enhance mutuality

Communication barriers
Self-concept disturbance
Absence of available significant others or peers
Limited physical mobility
Therapeutic isolation
Sociocultural dissonance
Environmental barriers
Altered thought processes

Defining characteristics

Verbalized or observed discomfort in social situations
Verbalized or observed inability to receive or communicate a satisfying sense of belonging, caring, interest, or shared history
Observed use of unsuccessful social interaction behaviors
Dysfunctional interaction with peers, family, and/or others
Family report of change in style or pattern of interaction

Social isolation   Aloneness experienced by an individual and perceived as imposed by others and as a negative or threatened state.

Related factors

Factors contributing to the absence of satisfying personal relationships, such as the following:
Delay in accomplishing developmental tasks
Immature interests
Alterations in physical appearance
Alterations in mental status
Unaccepted social behavior
Unaccepted social values
Altered state of wellness
Inadequate personal resources
Inability to engage in satisfying personal relationships

Defining characteristics

Objective
Absence of supportive significant other(s)—family, friends, group
Sad, dull affect
Inappropriate or immature interests and activities for developmental age or stage
Uncommunicative, withdrawn; no eye contact
Preoccupation with own thoughts; repetitive, meaningless actions
Projects hostility in voice, behavior

Seeks to be alone or exists in subculture

Evidence of physical and/or mental handicap or altered state of wellness

Shows behavior unaccepted by dominant cultural group

Subjective

Expresses feeling of aloneness imposed by others

Expresses feelings of rejection

Experiences feelings of indifference of others

Expresses values acceptable to subculture but is unable to accept values of dominant culture

Inadequacy in or absence of significant purpose in life

Inability to meet expectations of others

Insecurity in public

Expresses interests inappropriate to developmental age or stage

Spiritual distress (distress of the human spirit)   Disruption in the life principle that pervades a person's entire being and that integrates and transcends one's biological and psychosocial nature.

Related factors

Separation from religious and cultural ties

Challenged belief and value system (e.g., result of moral or ethical implications of therapy or result of intense suffering)

Defining characteristics

Expresses concern with meaning of life and death and/or belief systems

Anger toward God (as defined by the person)

Questions meaning of suffering

Verbalizes inner conflict about beliefs

Verbalizes concern about relationship with deity

Questions meaning of own existence

Inability to choose or chooses not to participate in usual religious practices

Seeks spiritual assistance

Questions moral and ethical implications of therapeutic regimen

Displacement of anger toward religious representatives

Description of nightmares or sleep disturbances

Alteration in behavior or mood evidenced by anger, crying, withdrawal, preoccupation, anxiety, hostility, apathy, etc.

Regards illness as punishment
Does not experience that God is forgiving
Inability to accept self
Engages in self-blame
Denies responsibilities for problems
Description of somatic complaints

Suffocation, high risk for   Accentuated risk of accidental suffocation (inadequate air available for inhalation).

Risk factors

Internal (individual) factors
  Reduced olfactory sensation
  Reduced motor abilities
  Lack of safety education
  Lack of safety precautions
  Cognitive or emotional difficulties
  Disease or injury process
External (environmental) factors
  Pillow placed in infant's crib
  Vehicle warming in closed garage
  Children playing with plastic bags or inserting small objects
    into their mouths or noses
  Discarded or unused refrigerators or freezers without doors
    removed
  Children left unattended in bathtubs or pools
  Household gas leaks
  Smoking in bed
  Use of fuel-burning heaters not vented to outside
  Low-strung clothesline
  Pacifer hung around infant's head
  Eating of large mouthfuls of food
  Propped bottle placed in infant's crib

Swallowing, impaired   The state in which an individual has decreased ability to voluntarily pass fluids and/or solids from the mouth to the stomach.

Related factors

Neuromuscular impairment (e.g., decreased or absent gag reflex, decreased strength or excursion of muscles involved in mastication, perceptual impairment, facial paralysis)
Mechanical obstruction (e.g., edema, tracheotomy tube, tumor)

Fatigue

Limited awareness

Reddened, irritated oropharyngeal cavity

Defining characteristics

Observed evidence of difficulty in swallowing (e.g., stasis of food in oral cavity, cough/choking)

Evidence of aspiration

Thermoregulation, ineffective
The state in which an individual's temperature fluctuates between hypothermia and hyperthermia.

Related factors

Trauma or illness

Immaturity

Aging

Fluctuating environmental temperature

Defining characteristics

Fluctuations in body temperature above or below normal range

See also defining characteristics of hypothermia and hyperthermia

Thought processes, altered
The state in which an individual experiences a disruption in cognitive operations and activities.

Related factors

Physiological changes

Psychological conflicts

Loss of memory

Impaired judgment

Sleep deprivation

Defining characteristics

Inaccurate interpretation of environment

Cognitive dissonance

Distractibility

Memory deficit or problems

Egocentricity

Hypervigilance/hypovigilance

Decreased ability to grasp ideas

Impaired ability to make decisions

Impaired ability to problem solve

Impaired ability to reason

Impaired ability to abstract or conceptualize

Impaired ability to calculate
Altered attention span—distractibility
Obsessions
Inability to follow commands
Disorientation to time, place, person, circumstances, and events
Changes in remote, recent, or immediate memory
Delusions
Ideas of reference
Hallucinations
Confabulation
Inappropriate social behavior
Altered sleep patterns
Inappropriate affect

Other possible defining characteristic

Inappropriate/nonreality-based thinking

Tissue integrity, impaired The state in which an individual experiences damage to mucous membrane or corneal, integumentary, or subcutaneous tissue. See also Oral Mucous Membrane, Altered.

Related factors

Altered circulation
Nutritional deficit/excess
Fluid deficit/excess
Knowledge deficit
Impaired physical mobility
Irritants
  Chemical (including body excretions, secretions, medications)
  Thermal (temperature extremes)
  Mechanical (pressure, shear, friction)
  Radiation (including therapeutic radiation)

Defining characteristics

Damaged or destroyed tissue (cornea, mucous membrane, integumentary, or subcutaneous)

Tissue perfusion, altered (specify type) (renal, cerebral, cardiopulmonary, gastrointestinal, peripheral) The state in which an individual experiences a decrease in nutrition and oxygenation at the cellular level due to a deficit in capillary blood supply.

Related factors
Interruption of flow, arterial
Interruption of flow, venous
Exchange problems
Hypervolemia
Hypovolemia
Defining characteristics
Skin temperature: cold extremities
Skin color
  Dependent, blue or purple
  Pale on elevation, and color does not return on lowering
    leg
  Diminished arterial pulsations
Skin quality: shining
Lack of lanugo
Round scars covered with atrophied skin
Gangrene
Slow-growing, dry, thick, brittle nails
Claudication
Blood pressure changes in extremities
Bruits
Slow healing of lesions

Trauma, high risk for   Accentuated risk of accidental tissue
injury (e.g., wound, burn, fracture)

Risk factors
Internal (individual) factors
  Weakness
  Poor vision
  Balancing difficulties
  Reduced temperature and/or tactile sensation
  Reduced large—or small—muscle coordination
  Reduced hand-eye coordination
  Lack of safety education
  Lack of safety precautions
  Insufficient finances to purchase safety equipment or effect
    repairs
  Cognitive or emotional difficulties
  History of previous trauma
External (environmental) factors
  Slippery floors (e.g., wet or highly waxed)
  Snow or ice on stairs, walkways
  Unanchored rugs

Bathtub without hand grip or antislip equipment

Use of unsteady ladder or chairs

Entering unlighted rooms

Unsturdy or absent stair rails

Unanchored electric wires

Litter or liquid spills on floors or stairways

High beds

Children playing without gates at top of stairs

Obstructed passageways

Unsafe window protection in homes with young children

Inappropriate call-for-aid mechanisms for bed-resting client

Pot handles facing toward front of stove

Bathing in very hot water (e.g., unsupervised bathing of young children)

Potential igniting of gas leaks

Delayed lighting of gas burner or oven

Experimenting with chemicals or gasoline

Unscreened fires or heaters

Wearing of plastic aprons or flowing clothing around open flame

Children playing with matches, candles, cigarettes

Inadequately stored combustibles or corrosives (e.g., matches, oily rags, lye)

Highly flammable children's toys or clothing

Overloaded fuse boxes

Contact with rapidly moving machinery, industrial belts, or pulleys

Sliding on coarse bed linen or struggling within bed restraints

Faulty electrical plugs, frayed wires, or defective appliances

Contact with acids or alkalis

Playing with fireworks or gunpowder

Contact with intense cold

Overexposure to sun, sun lamps, radiotherapy

Use of cracked dishware or glasses

Knives stored uncovered

Guns or ammunition stored unlocked

Large icicles hanging from roof

Exposure to dangerous machinery

Children playing with sharp-edged toys

High-crime neighborhood and vulnerable patient

Driving a mechanically unsafe vehicle

Driving after partaking of alcoholic beverages or drugs
Driving at excessive speeds
Driving without necessary visual aids
Children riding in front seat of car
Smoking in bed or near oxygen
Overloaded electrical outlets
Grease waste collected on stoves
Use of thin or worn pot holders or mitts
Unrestrained babies riding in car
Nonuse or misuse of seat restraints
Nonuse or misuse of necessary headgear for motorized
cyclists or young children carried on adult bicycles
Unsafe road or road-crossing conditions
Play or work near vehicle pathways (e.g., driveways, lanes,
railroad tracks)

Unilateral neglect
The state in which an individual is perceptually unaware of and inattentive to one side of the body.

Related factors
Effects of disturbed perceptual abilities (e.g., hemianopsia)
One-sided blindness
Neurological illness or trauma
Defining characteristics
Consistent inattention to stimuli on affected side
Inadequate self-care
Positioning and/or safety precautions in regard to affected
side
Does not look toward affected side
Leaves food on plate on affected side

Urinary elimination, altered
The state in which an individual experiences a disturbance in urine elimination. See also Incontinence (functional, reflex, stress, total, urge).

Related factors
Sensory motor impairment
Neuromuscular impairment
Mechanical trauma
Defining characteristics
Dysuria
Frequency
Hesitancy
Incontinence

Nocturia
Retention
Urgency

Urinary retention   The state in which an individual experiences incomplete emptying of the bladder.

Related factors
High urethral pressure caused by weak detrusor
Inhibition of reflex arc
Strong sphincter
Blockage
Defining characteristics
Bladder distention
Small, frequent voiding or absence of urine output
Sensation of bladder fullness
Dribbling
Residual urine
Dysuria
Overflow incontinence

Ventilation, inability to sustain spontaneous   A state in which the response pattern of decreased energy reserves results in an individual's inability to maintain breathing adequate to support life.

Related factors
Metabolic factors
Respiratory muscle fatigue
Defining characteristics
Major
Dyspnea
Increased metabolic rate
Minor
Increased restlessness
Apprehension
Increased use of accessory muscles
Decreased tidal volume
Increased heart rate
Decreased po_2 level
Increased pco_2 level
Decreased cooperation
Decreased Sao_2 level

Ventilatory weaning response, dysfunctional
(DVWR) A state in which an individual cannot adjust to low-ered levels of mechanical ventilator support, which interrupts and prolongs the weaning process.

Related factors
Physical
Ineffective airway clearance
Sleep pattern disturbance
Inadequate nutrition
Uncontrolled pain or discomfort
Psychological
Knowledge deficit of the weaning process/patient role
Patient-perceived inefficacy about the ability to wean
Decreased motivation
Decreased self-esteem
Anxiety: moderate, severe
Fear
Hopelessness
Powerlessness
Insufficient trust in the nurse
Situational
Uncontrolled episodic energy demands or problems
Inappropriate pacing of diminished ventilator support
Inadequate social support
Adverse environment (noisy, active environment; negative events in the room; low nurse-patient ratio; extended nurse absence from bedside; unfamiliar nursing staff)
History of ventilator dependence >1 week
History of multiple unsuccessful weaning attempts

Defining characteristics
Mild DVWR
Major
Responds to lowered levels of mechanical ventilator support with the following:
Restlessness
Slight increased respiratory rate from baseline
Minor
Responds to lowered levels of mechanical ventilator support with the following:
Expressed feelings of increased need for oxygen; breathing discomfort; fatigue; warmth
Queries about possible machine malfunction
Increased concentration on breathing

Moderate DVWR

Major

Responds to lowered levels of mechanical ventilator support with the following:

Slight increase from baseline blood pressure <20mm Hg

Slight increase from baseline heart rate <20 beats/minute

Baseline increase in respiratory rate <5 breaths/minute

Minor

Hypervigilance to activities

Inability to respond to coaching

Inability to cooperate

Apprehension

Diaphoresis

Eye widening

Decreased air entry on auscultation

Color changes; pale; slight cyanosis

Slight respiratory accessory muscle use

Severe DVWR

Major

Responds to lowered levels of mechanical ventilator support with the following:

Agitation

Deterioration in arterial blood gas levels from current baseline

Increase from baseline blood pressure >20mm Hg

Increase from baseline heart rate >20 beats/minute

Respiratory rate increases significantly from baseline

Minor

Profuse diaphoresis

Full respiratory accessory muscle use

Shallow, gasping breaths

Paradoxical abdominal breathing

Discoordinated breathing with the ventilator

Decreased level of consciousness

Adventitious breath sounds, audible airway secretions

Cyanosis

Violence, high risk for: self-directed or directed at others
The state in which an individual experiences behaviors that can be physically harmful either to the self or others.

Risk factors

Antisocial character

Battered women

68

VIOLENCE, HIGH RISK FOR: SELF-DIRECTED OR DIRECTED AT OTHERS

Catatonic excitement
Child abuse
Manic excitement
Organic brain syndrome
Panic states
Rage reactions
Suicidal behavior
Temporal lobe epilepsy
Toxic reactions to medication

Nursing diagnoses: prototype care plans

ACTIVITY INTOLERANCE

Activity Intolerance

Related factors: Ineffective pain management; imbalance between oxygen supply and demand*

Audrey M. McLane, Linda K. Young, Marie McGuire, and Marilyn Harter

PATIENT GOALS/ EXPECTED OUTCOMES	NURSING INTERVENTIONS/ SCIENTIFIC RATIONALE
Develop activity/rest pattern consistent with physiological limitations as evidenced by the following:	
Exercise log indicates patient maintains activity level at 4 mets or less	Assist patient in identifying factors that decrease/increase activity tolerance. *Accurate assessment of factors that decrease/increase activity tolerance provides the foundation for effective care planning.*
Monitors physiological response to activity	Develop individualized activity/ exercise program, inclusive of home exercise program. *Individualized programs of physical activity have beneficial effects on cardiac performance.*
Modifies activity that produces pain	
Tolerates job-related activities without pain or fatigue	Discuss necessity to pace activities. *Pacing activity levels lessens the demands of cardiac workload.*
Develops strategies to take medications according to plan	Collaborate with patient to tailor medication taking to demands of activities. *Taking medications as prescribed can enhance activity tolerance.*
Engages in regular exercise (i.e., 4 mets or less)	
	Teach patient to monitor physiological response to activity (e.g., pulse rate, shortness of breath). *Monitoring facilitates evaluation of the activity level for daily living.*
	Teach patient to eliminate/reduce activities that provoke pain or fatigue.

*Myocardial infarction [MI] patient nearing discharge from acute care.

Activity Intolerance—cont'd

PATIENT GOALS/ EXPECTED OUTCOMES	NURSING INTERVENTIONS/ *SCIENTIFIC RATIONALE*
	Teach patient warning signs of cardiac decompensation.
	Teach patient use of exercise log to record exercise activities and responses (e.g., pulse, shortness of breath, anxiety). *Logging may increase compliance.*
Makes appointment with physician for evaluation of activity intolerance	Refer to physician for evaluation of therapeutic regimen.
Recognize influences of emotional responses on exercise tolerance as evidenced by the following:	
Learns/practices relaxation techniques	Teach patient/significant other influence of fear/anxiety as it relates to activity tolerance. *Fear and anxiety may enhance activity intolerance.*
Patient/significant other creates private, quiet place in home for patient to practice relaxation techniques	
Significant other understands reason for, and use of, patient's cognitive coping strategies	Teach cognitive coping strategies (e.g., imagery, relaxation, controlled breathing). *Emotional responses to activity intolerance may be effectively managed through use of cognitive coping strategies.*
	Encourage significant other to learn coping strategies and/or assist by guiding/coaching practice of controlled breathing.
	Teach significant other to help patient pace activities. *Social support enhances compliance.*
Use social support network to maintain desired life-style as evidenced by the following:	

continued.

ACTIVITY INTOLERANCE

PATIENT GOALS/ EXPECTED OUTCOMES	NURSING INTERVENTIONS/ *SCIENTIFIC RATIONALE*
Significant other assists with activities of daily living (ADLs) to prevent activity level from exceeding 4 mets	Collaborate with patient/significant other to establish plan of daily activities consistent with desired life-style which require <4 mets. *Achieving and maintaining a vital and productive life while remaining within the heart's ability to respond to increases in activity and stress is individualized for patients.*
Friends/neighbors help with home maintenance activities (e.g., lawn mowing, putting up storm windows) Patient/significant other prepares priority list of desired recreational activities	Encourage patient/significant other to seek assistance with home maintenance activities from friends/neighbors. *Social support helps enhance recovery and maintain a desired life-style.* Determine interest of patient/significant other in sexual counseling. *Sexual activity is often a great concern to patients and their sexual partners.*

References 11, 102, 141, 177, 266, 412, 478, 551.

Activity Intolerance, High Risk for

Risk factors: Fatigue/weakness; does not comply with exercise prescription; >15% overweight*
Audrey M. McLane, Linda K. Young, Marilyn Harter, and Marie McGuire

PATIENT GOALS/ EXPECTED OUTCOMES	NURSING INTERVENTIONS/ *SCIENTIFIC RATIONALE*
Participate in cardiac reha- bilitation program as evi- denced by the following:	
Attends informational classes for all post–myocardial infarc- tion patients	Encourage/negotiate with pa- tient to participate in cardiac rehabilitation program. *Car- diac rehabilitation programs can facilitate the patient's ability to achieve and main- tain a vital and productive life while remaining within the heart's ability to respond to increases in activity and stress.*
Makes decision to enroll in postdischarge cardiac rehabili- tation program	Assist patient in verbalizing anxiety/fear/concerns about engaging in exercise. *Recog- nizing fear and anxiety is the first step to managing them.*
Patient/spouse clarifies values with nurse's assistance	Assist patient with clarification of values. *Becoming aware of one's own values may enhance compliance with prescribed regime.*
Verbalizes fears about increas- ing level of activity	Provide written specifications for duration, intensity, fre- quency, and mets level of ADLs and recreational activi- ties. *Specific data about toler- ance of ADLs and recreational activities promote safe func- tioning.*

*For the patient after myocardial infarction (NYHA Classification I). NYHA New York Heart Association Functional Classification of Heart Disease Class I—No lim-itations. Ordinary physical activity does not cause undue fatigue, dyspnea, or pal-pitation. *continued.*

PATIENT GOALS/ EXPECTED OUTCOMES	NURSING INTERVENTIONS/ *SCIENTIFIC RATIONALE*
Integrate exercise prescription into ADLs by the following:	
Experiences less fatigue/weakness after exercise regimen	Teach patient/spouse benefits of exercise regimen in decreasing fatigue/weakness.
Uses exercise log to record distance walked and symptoms experienced	Teach patient/spouse use of exercise log to record activities, time, duration, intensity, and physiological responses (e.g., pulse rate, shortness of breath, lightheadedness). *Logging may increase compliance.*
Uses written list of activities with met levels to guide activities	
Uses conservation techniques for household tasks to have energy available for desired activities	Teach self-monitoring of heart rate during exercise. *Self-monitoring promotes self-care.*
	Teach self-evaluation of response to activity, including actions for specific signs and symptoms.
	Teach patient long-term value of increased activity. *Highlighting positive long-term effects may increase compliance.*
	Encourage spouse to accompany patient on walks. *Social support may enhance participation in this activity.*

Activity Intolerance, High Risk for—cont'd

PATIENT GOALS/ EXPECTED OUTCOMES	NURSING INTERVENTIONS/ SCIENTIFIC RATIONALE
Gradually reduce body weight as evidenced by the following:	
Agrees to consult with dietitian to begin weight reduction program	Negotiate with patient to make decision to lose weight. *Client input and motivation are factors affecting patient participation in weight reduction.* Collaborate with dietitian to provide low-calorie snacks and diet sodas. *Predetermined low-caloric meals help increase the likelihood of limited caloric intake.*
Prepares shopping list for low-calorie foods with spouse	Assist patient/spouse with preparing shopping list for low-calorie meals.
Disposes of high-calorie snacks kept at bedside	
Instructs spouse to dispose of high-calorie snacks in cupboards at home	
Sets realistic weekly weight-loss goal.	Refer to dietitian for diet instruction and for recommending caloric requirements.
Achieves desired body weight	Monitor weight twice a week to *help patient realize weight loss and gain, which can reinforce changed behavior.*

References 102, 141, 177, 207, 266, 395, 451, 478, 551.

Adjustment, Impaired

Related factors: Disability requiring change in life-style;
altered locus of control.*
Elizabeth Kelchner Gerety and Gertrude K. McFarland

PATIENT GOALS/ EXPECTED OUTCOMES	NURSING INTERVENTIONS/ *SCIENTIFIC RATIONALE*
Modify life-style to decrease disability and experience maximal control and independence within limits imposed by changed health status as evidenced by the following:	
Recognizes that choice of self-care practices can influence adjustment to disability	Provide opportunity for expression of fears related to MI and potential physical limitations.
Demonstrates self-care practices that are within prescribed treatment regimen	Assist patient in working through emotional responses to MI (e.g., denial, anxiety, or depression).
Makes future plans that are congruent with changed health status.	Encourage identification of personal strengths and intact roles *to maximize sense of ability for regaining control.*
Uses strengths and potentials to engage in maximally independent and constructive life-style	Provide information about illness and what to expect during hospitalization, based on assessment of learning readiness. *Such strategies reinforce positive psychological and social outcomes and reduce fear and anxiety associated with the hospitalization.*
	Assist patient to select self-care practices that enhance adjustment to disability (e.g., maintaining balanced exercise/rest regimen).

*For the patient following myocardial infarction.

Adjustment, Impaired—cont'd

PATIENT GOALS/ EXPECTED OUTCOMES	NURSING INTERVENTIONS/ SCIENTIFIC RATIONALE
	Teach patient and family to differentiate between denial of the presence of change in health status and denial of possible limitations.
	Generate hope by assisting patient to identify previous coping behaviors and support systems used for past problem solving.
	Collaborate with patient and other staff *to assist in determining what will aid in control and management of patient's health status change.*
	Encourage patient to use problem-focused coping strategies by enabling patient to discuss own health problems with others in a similar situation and providing adequate information about the illness. *Patients using problem-focused coping strategies and perceived self-control appear to have less psychosocial difficulty with post-MI adjustment.*
	Actively include family and significant others in entire cardiac rehabilitation process. *The perceived beliefs of significant others are important for patient's adherence to medical regimen.*
	Facilitate compromise when patient's identified goals differ from goals developed by health-care providers or from family expectations.

continued.

ADJUSTMENT, IMPAIRED

PATIENT GOALS/ EXPECTED OUTCOMES	NURSING INTERVENTIONS/ SCIENTIFIC RATIONALE
	Encourage patient to maintain a sense of control (within physical limitations) by making decisions related to specific aspects of care, sharing observations of physical status and progress with caregivers, and assuming responsibility for selected aspects of care.
	Assess for possible correlation between family's willingness to support patient's changed life-style and patient's ability to adapt to disability.
	Facilitate discussion by patient and family of topics that are not related to disability (e.g., current events, family activities, hobbies, recreational interests).
Assume responsibility for using social resources for assistance in ongoing health management as evidenced by the following: Uses available health-care system and community resources	Consistently convey value of self-directive behavior on patient's part.
	Encourage patient and family to explore such resources as Medicare, Social Security, and disability insurance.
	Refer patient and family to community resources, such as cardiac support groups or the American Heart Association for assistance with ongoing informational needs, advocacy issues, and current developments in treatment and research.

References 45, 83, 93, 181, 278, 285, 314, 400, 564.

Airway Clearance, Ineffective

Related factors: Ineffective coughing; excessive secretions with intubated trachea*
Mi Ja Kim and Mary V. Hanley

PATIENT GOALS/ EXPECTED OUTCOMES	NURSING INTERVENTIONS/ *SCIENTIFIC RATIONALE*
Remove secretions more effectively as evidenced by the following: Secretions are minimally expectorated or suctioned Breath sounds are clear after treatments Tracheal tube is free of plugs Patient or significant other is able to perform airway clearance procedures	Assist and teach patient to cough after several deep breaths. Help patient to assume a comfortable cough position (e.g., high-Fowler's with knees bent and a lightweight pillow over abdomen to augment expiratory pressures and minimize discomfort). *Effective cough requires a deep breath and contraction of expiratory muscles, especially the abdominal muscles, to increase the intrathoracic pressure and expel secretions.* Remove expectorated secretions from opening of tracheotomy tube using aseptic technique. Use clean technique in home. Note volume, viscosity, and color of secretions. Teach patient alternate cough techniques (e.g., huff or quad) if patient is having difficulty with above method. Avoid deep suctioning; if patient can cough secretions to tracheal tube, suction the tube only. Perform chest physical therapy maneuvers to drain remote areas of lung by gravity (add percussion, if not contraindicated).

continued.

PATIENT GOALS/ EXPECTED OUTCOMES	NURSING INTERVENTIONS/ SCIENTIFIC RATIONALE
	Vibrate area of interest during exhalation; be prepared to collect expectorated secretions or suction as described below. *Chest physical therapy consists of vibration, percussion, and postural drainage of selected lung units (e.g., segments). Vibration applied to chest wall, together with gravity and slow exhalation after deep breathing, dislodges retained secretions from the underlying airways and facilitates mucus clearance.*
	Initiate cough assists (as described previously) or provide a fast Ambu breath to stimulate cough receptors. Quickly release hand pressure on bag and again be ready to collect secretions.
	Adjust frequency of therapy according to achievement of outcome criteria, target times, and patient comfort.
	Provide systemic hydration, which is calculated from patient's intake, output, and body weight. *The usual water loss from expired gas is 30 ml per day, depending on respiratory rate and route of inspiration. Systemic dehydration or excess adversely affects the mucociliary escalator (i.e., relationship of cilia, sol, and gel layers) and impairs mucociliary clearance.*

Airway Clearance, Ineffective—cont'd

PATIENT GOALS/ EXPECTED OUTCOMES	NURSING INTERVENTIONS/ *SCIENTIFIC RATIONALE*
	Provide humidified gas at 37° C and 100% saturation ventilator, T-piece connector attached to wide-bore tubing or tracheostomy mask. *Inspired gas is normally filtered, warmed, and humidified by the upper airway, primarily the nose. By the time the inspired gas reaches the trachea, it is 37° C and 100% humidifed. When the normal host defenses are bypassed, drier and cooler air dehydrates the respiratory mucous membranes, impairs mucociliary clearance, and causes inspissated tracheobronchial secretions.*
	Remove condensed vapor from inspiratory line prn and change humidifier, connectors, and tubing every day.
	Protect opening of tracheal tube from unfiltered ambient air and avoid introduction of foreign objects and blind instillation of fluids (e.g., saline).
	Perform intratracheal suctioning only when secretions are reachable by catheter and patient cannot effectively cough. Prepare patient for this uncomfortable and potentially traumatic procedure and explain purpose and sequence of maneuvers.

continued.

AIRWAY CLEARANCE, INEFFECTIVE

PATIENT GOALS/ EXPECTED OUTCOMES	NURSING INTERVENTIONS/ *SCIENTIFIC RATIONALE*
	Use aseptic technique during suctioning; clean technique is appropriate in home.
	Preoxygenate with 100% oxygen before suctioning.
	If patient is spontaneously breathing and has a dominant hypoxic drive to breathe, adjust Fio_2 level accordingly.
	After preoxygenation and hyperinflations, use a sterile catheter that is one half the diameter of tube and apply intermittent negative pressure for less than 15 seconds per pass; reoxygenate and remain with patient until return to baseline vital signs. *Suctioning removes air as well as secretions from the airways and induces hypoxemia.*
	Use minimal cuff inflation. If patient is spontaneously breathing and can swallow oropharyngeal secretions and oral feedings without aspiration, the cuff can be left deflated to minimize tracheal damage.
	Consult physician for adjunct therapies and further assessment, mucolytics, bronchodilators, antibiotics, fiberoptic bronchoscopy, and diagnostic tests (e.g., sputum for culture, sensitivity and Gram stain, chest x-ray examination).
	Teach patient or significant other airway clearance procedure and administration of medical adjunctive therapies, as appropriate.

References 59, 107, 231, 232, 297, 340, 352, 354, 473, 530, 588.

Anxiety

Related factor: Unmet needs
Gertrude K. McFarland and Thelma I. Bates

PATIENT GOALS/ EXPECTED OUTCOMES	NURSING INTERVENTIONS/ *SCIENTIFIC RATIONALE*
Experience reduced anxiety level as evidenced by the following: Demonstrates decreased tension, apprehension, perspiration, insomnia, restlessness, hand tremors, quivering voice, perceptual distortions, and desire to harm self.	Monitor level of anxiety through observation of patient's state of alertness, ability to comprehend, problem-solving ability, ability to be redirected, narrowing perceptual field, focused or scattered attention, level of intellectual functioning, ability to manage ADLs, and appropriateness of response to situation. Maintain calm and safe environment by decreasing stimuli, talking to and reassuring patient, and removing harmful objects if necessary. *Structure in the environment can assist the patient in decreasing level of anxiety.* Encourage involvement in activities, depending on level of anxiety. Guide participation in self-care. Assist patient in identifying possible sources of stress along with use of alcohol, caffeine, nicotine, and other drugs. *Chemical substances can influence anxiety level.*

continued.

Anxiety—cont'd

ANXIETY

PATIENT GOALS/ EXPECTED OUTCOMES	NURSING INTERVENTIONS/ *SCIENTIFIC RATIONALE*
Demonstrates increased ability to discuss and monitor own behavior, identify stressors, and become more involved in activities and initiating interactions with peers.	Help patient to connect behavior with feelings by encouraging patient to discuss feelings, obtaining patient's perception of anxiety experienced, helping patient to identify how anxiety is manifested through behavior, and exploring with patient ways of anticipating anxiety. *Assists patient in gaining awareness and understanding of the relationship between anxiety level and behavior and in participating in managing own care.*

Demonstrate effective coping skills as evidenced by the following:
Able to problem solve
Demonstrate relaxation techniques
Able to meet self-care needs
Able to form interpersonal relationships
	Explore coping mechanisms with patient; help patient to identify those coping mechanisms which were successful in decreasing anxiety.
	Help patient to identify adaptive coping mechanisms within patient's own cultural expectations.
	Discuss importance of regular exercise program.
	Review problem-solving process (e.g., organize, prioritize, implement, evaluate, and teach relaxation techniques).
	Instruct in deep breathing.
	   Instruct patient to take slow, deep breaths (eyes may be opened or closed).
	   Repeat and demonstrate as necessary.

Anxiety—cont'd

PATIENT GOALS/ EXPECTED OUTCOMES	NURSING INTERVENTIONS/ *SCIENTIFIC RATIONALE*
	Teach use of progressive relaxation *to prevent or reduce level of existing anxiety.*
	Tell patient to sit or lie in a comfortable position in a quiet area (Patient should close eyes unless doing so makes him/her uncomfortable.)
	At periods throughout exercise, ask patient to focus on breathing (slow and deep).
	To begin exercise, instruct patient to get in a comfortable position and imagine being in a quiet, comfortable place (e.g., on a beach, listening to a gentle rain). Then instruct patient to tense gently (for 5 seconds and without injury) and then relax each muscle group (10 to 15 seconds).
	Begin with toes and feet and move progressively upward—calf, thigh, buttock, lower back, hands (make fist), lower arm, upper arm, shoulders, neck, and ending with face (grimace). After relaxing face, patient should remain quiet for 15 minutes (or as patient can tolerate), concentrating on peace, quiet, and breathing.
	Instruct patient to use entire exercise or just for areas of tension.

References 141, 178, 283, 453, 542, 562, 622.

Aspiration, High Risk for

Risk factor: Enteral feeding via nasogastric/nasointestinal tubes*

Kathryn Hennessy and Mi Ja Kim

PATIENT GOALS/ EXPECTED OUTCOMES	NURSING INTERVENTIONS/ *SCIENTIFIC RATIONALE*
Experience no aspiration as evidenced by the following:	
No gastric distention; normal bowel sounds	Orient patient and teach significant other about expected procedure for enteral feeding via nasogastric tube.
No complaints of nausea or vomiting	Confirm tube placement after insertion and at regular intervals at least every 4 hours with continuous feeding or before each intermittent feeding.
Vital signs within normal limits for patient	Confirm initial tube placement by chest x-ray examination in collaboration with physician.
	Aspirate stomach contents. If needed, check aspirate for acidic pH level to confirm initial tube placement. *An acidic pH indicates that the nasogastric tube is in the stomach.* If the tube becomes dislodged after feedings are initiated, check for presence of glucose. *The presence of glucose in the secretions reflects the presence of tube feeding formula in the stomach. Glucose is not present in tracheal or pulmonary secretions.*

*For the patient who has a decreased level of consciousness as a result of severe trauma.

Aspiration, High Risk for—cont'd

PATIENT GOALS/ EXPECTED OUTCOMES	NURSING INTERVENTIONS/ SCIENTIFIC RATIONALE
	If aspiration of stomach contents is difficult, the injection of 10 cc of air before aspiration may prevent tube from collapsing during aspiration. *Positioning patient on the right side helps to pool secretions, thus making it easier to obtain gastric contents when aspirating through a small-bore feeding tube.* Monitor other potential risk factors, such as decreased level of consciousness and sedated state. Be aware that coughing, vomiting, and suctioning may dislodge feeding tube. Tape feeding tube securely and monitor tube markings for possible tube migration every 4 hours and before each feeding. Assess for gastric retention every 4 hours through the following procedures: Check gastric residuals. If residuals are 50% greater than prescribed volume, hold tube feeding and recheck residual in 1 hour; notify physician if this occurs for two consecutive measurements of residuals (tube feedings may need to be discontinued).

Continued

PATIENT GOALS/ EXPECTED OUTCOMES	NURSING INTERVENTIONS/ *SCIENTIFIC RATIONALE*
	Check abdominal girths serially. Measure from one anterior iliac crest to the other. An increase of 8 to 10 cm above baseline should be considered significant, and tube feeding should be stopped and physician notified. Evaluate gastric motility at least every 4 hours through the following procedures: 　Auscultate bowel sounds. 　Percuss abdomen for air. 　Assess for nausea/vomiting. 　Assess for diarrhea/constipation. 　Assess for gastric distention. 　If bowel sounds are absent, distention is present, and/or there is nausea/vomiting, hold the tube feedings and notify the physician. *The absence of bowel sounds with abdominal distention and nausea and/or vomiting may indicate a paralytic ileus and thus contraindicate tube feedings.* Maintain proper patient positioning during tube feeding administration through the following procedures: 　Increase head of bed 30 to 45 degrees during feeding to minimize amount of feeding in stomach.

Aspiration, High Risk for—cont'd

PATIENT GOALS/ EXPECTED OUTCOMES	NURSING INTERVENTIONS/ *SCIENTIFIC RATIONALE*
	If unable to elevate head of bed, turn patient to *right side to facilitate passage of stomach contents through pylorus. The side lying position also allows emesis to drain from the mouth rather than be aspirated into the lungs.* (When side lying is not possible, consider an alternate feeding method.) Stop tube feeding 30 to 60 minutes before physical activity and procedures that require lowering of patient's head.
	Monitor patient for signs of aspiration (cyanosis, dyspnea, cough, wheezing, tachycardia, fever, massive atelectasis with pulmonary edema, hypoxemia, temperature greater than 38° C for 24 hours).
	Check vital signs, temperature every 4 to 8 hours.
	Auscultate breath sounds every 4 to 8 hours.
	Observe and record color and character of sputum every 8 hours. (Add blue food coloring to tube feeding). *The presence of blue food coloring in the pulmonary secretions indicates that tube feeding has been aspirated. Blue food coloring may cause false positive hemoccult readings for stool.*

continued.

Aspiration, High Risk for—cont'd

PATIENT GOALS/ EXPECTED OUTCOMES	NURSING INTERVENTIONS/ *SCIENTIFIC RATIONALE*
	Check pulmonary-tracheal secretions for glucose with reagent strip every 4 to 8 hours (in high-risk patients). *Positive glucose indicates presence of formula in pulmonary secretions (false-positive may occur with presence of blood in pulmonary secretions).*

References 36, 71, 303, 361, 392, 411, 499, 590.

Body Image Disturbance

Related factor: Difficulty accepting body image*
Gertrude K. McFarland and Karen E. Inaba

PATIENT GOALS/ EXPECTED OUTCOMES	NURSING INTERVENTIONS/ *SCIENTIFIC RATIONALE*
Accept body change and incorporate into self-concept so as to maintain a positive body image as evidenced by the following: Makes positive statements about body image Personalizes loss of body part Looks at or touches affected body part Expresses acceptance of altered body image Uses available resources for information and support	Assess patient's current perceptions and feelings about mastectomy and resulting body image change. Assess patient's perception of impact of mastectomy on relationship with spouse or significant other *to identify distortions*. Respect patient's need for a period of withdrawal or denial *to minimize intrusiveness and increased vulnerability*. Assist patient in expressing feelings about loss, *in order to support normal grieving*. Provide information about cosmetic aids and use of clothing styles *to improve self-image*. Encourage participation in support services and groups in the community *to connect with peers for information and validation*. Praise constructive problem solving to enhance appearance *to reinforce adaptive behaviors*.

References 69, 79, 272, 424, 432, 474, 492, 496, 520.
*For the patient postmastectomy.

BODY TEMPERATURE, ALTERED, HIGH RISK FOR

Body Temperature, Altered, High Risk for

Risk factor: Trauma affecting hypothalamus*
Kathryn Czurylo and Mi Ja Kim

PATIENT GOALS/ EXPECTED OUTCOMES	NURSING INTERVENTIONS/ *SCIENTIFIC RATIONALE*
Maintain normothermia as evidenced by the following:	Monitor temperature every 2 hours or use continuous temperature monitoring.
No signs or symptoms of hyperthermia (e.g., flushing irritability, seizures)	Monitor other vital signs every 2 hours.
Normothermia	Administer steroids to decrease edema around area of hypothalamus as ordered.
Vital signs within normal limits for patient	Administer antipyretic agents as ordered.
Serum electrolyte levels and fluid balance within normal limits	Adjust environmental temperature to patient's needs if body temperature is altered.
	Adjust patient temperature if body temperature is altered, using cooling mattress and tepid baths as necessary. When using cooling mattress, bring temperature down gradually *to prevent shivering, which causes increased oxygen consumption.*
	Administer IV fluids at room temperature.
	Continue to monitor and report signs and symptoms of hyperthermia.
	Consider other causes of fever, including drug fever (check liver function studies) and infectious process (check CBC/ cultures).

References 64, 76, 134, 338, 404, 537.
*For the patient with a head injury.

Bowel Incontinence

Related factors: Inaccessibility of toilet facilities; anal sphincter damage

Audrey M. McLane and Ruth E. McShane

PATIENT GOALS/ EXPECTED OUTCOMES	NURSING INTERVENTIONS/ SCIENTIFIC RATIONALE
Establish a regular pattern of bowel elimination as evidenced by the following:	
Accepts use of commode	Collaborate with family member and patient to establish area for use of commode on first floor of residence.
Uses commode after all meals	Provide for privacy when using commode.
	Collaborate with family member to develop toileting routine after meals.
	Instruct family member to provide early morning breakfast to stimulate gastrocolic reflex.
Practices pelvic floor exercises with coaching from nurse and/ or family member	Teach patient pelvic floor exercises and coach practice sessions during each visit. *Pelvic floor exercises help to strengthen anal sphincters and may prevent episodes of incontinence.*
Episodes of bowel incontinence gradually decrease in frequency	Instruct patient to maintain contractions for 3 to 4 seconds and then repeat without tensing muscles of legs, buttocks, or abdomen. *If contractions are maintained for 1 minute, sphincters tend to fatigue and go into a refractory stage.*
	Collaborate with family member to arrange for home health aide to provide lunch and assist patient with toileting routine.
	Teach home health aide how to coach patient with pelvic floor exercises.

continued.

Bowel Incontinence—cont'd

BOWEL INCONTINENCE

PATIENT GOALS/ EXPECTED OUTCOMES	NURSING INTERVENTIONS/ *SCIENTIFIC RATIONALE*
Skin breakdown is prevented as evidenced by the following: Perirectal skin is normal in appearance	Teach family member to check rectal area daily for signs of redness. Provide patient/family member with written directions for daily skin care. Teach family member to monitor all medications, including nonprescription medications. Provide information about incontinence aids.
Social functioning is increased as evidenced by the following: Uses protective clothing Absence of fecal odor Participates in social activities at least twice a week	Plan with patient/family member for short trips away from home. Encourage use of continence aids. Demonstrate sensitivity to patient's feelings about odor and incontinence episodes.

References 9, 344, 349, 362, 378, 379.

Breastfeeding, Effective

Related factors: Appropriate knowledge; support sources
Pamela D. Hill and Mi Ja Kim

PATIENT GOALS/ EXPECTED OUTCOMES	NURSING INTERVENTIONS/ SCIENTIFIC RATIONALE
Adequate lactation is maintained as evidenced by the following: Infant demonstrates adequate weight gain appropriate to age Mother continues breastfeeding as long as intended	Review routine pattern of breastfeeding. *Knowledge of physiology of milk production is crucial in the management of lactation.* Reinforce previous knowledge of the breastfeeding process. Encourage frequent rest periods. *Fatigue may inhibit the let-down reflex.* Discuss nutritious diet of increased calories, protein, and vitamins. Instruct to avoid intentional weight loss. *Proper nutrition is necessary to maintain health of mother and infant and maintain adequate lactation.* Encourage to maintain adequate fluid intake and drink to satisfy thirst; discourage taking excessive fluids. *Forcing fluids negatively affects milk production.* Encourage mother to avoid use of cigarettes and birth control pills until lactation is well established. *Nicotine may decrease prolactin levels and inhibit let-down reflex. High dosage oral contraceptives may decrease milk volume by interfering with lactation.*

continued.

PATIENT GOALS/ EXPECTED OUTCOMES	NURSING INTERVENTIONS/ SCIENTIFIC RATIONALE
	Provide anticipatory guidance for infant developmental changes that affect breastfeeding (growth spurts at 2 to 3 weeks, 6 weeks, and 3 months). *Mother may misperceive an inadequate milk supply due to increased feedings of infant.*
	Avoid introducing solids until infant is 5 to 6 months of age. *Current recommendations stress delaying the addition of solids; solids may diminish milk supply.*
	Demonstrate how to express/ pump breastmilk and store properly. *Adequate stimulation of the breasts is necessary to maintain lactation when mother-infant are separated.*
	Offer praise and encouragement *to reinforce positive breastfeeding behavior.*
	Discuss with mother her feelings about breastfeeding outside the home.
Prevent breast complications as evidenced by the following: Mother develops no breast or nipple complications	Encourage use of supportive bra 24 hours a day. Advise how to choose correct bra and bra size. Bra should give support and not bind. Avoid underwires and elastic around the cups, *which may prevent sufficient drainage by pressing on milk ducts.*

Breastfeeding, Effective—cont'd

PATIENT GOALS/ EXPECTED OUTCOMES	NURSING INTERVENTIONS/ *SCIENTIFIC RATIONALE*
	Stress importance of preventing engorgement. *Engorgement of the breast can be painful, may predispose to the development of nipple fissures and breast abscesses, and is associated with lactation failure.*
	Encourage mother to use both breasts at a feeding. *Inadequate drainage of milk sinuses can lead to a diminished milk production.*
	Encourage mother to nurse at least 10 minutes/breast before switching. Allow adequate time for the let-down reflex to occur *to ensure that the infant receives the hindmilk and not only the low-calorie foremilk.*
	Demonstrate how to massage breasts during feeding. *Breast massage causes the hindmilk to move from the alveoli to the lactiferous sinuses, thus facilitating the let-down and emptying of the breasts.*
	Encourage mother to alternate infant's feeding positions. *Changing positions will help to alleviate stress on the nipples and minimize irritation.*
	Teach to avoid external pressure on breasts (e.g., positions that put pressure on one spot for long periods).
	Demonstrate how to empty breast manually or with pump if baby does not empty. *Ducts may become plugged and mastitis develop if breast is not emptied.*

continued.

BREASTFEEDING, EFFECTIVE

PATIENT GOALS/ EXPECTED OUTCOMES	NURSING INTERVENTIONS/ SCIENTIFIC RATIONALE
Maintain family adaptation to breastfeeding process as evidenced by the following:	
Family members verbalize comfortableness with the mother's breastfeeding	Provide age-appropriate literature about breastfeeding to family members. *Support and encouragement from the male partner and family significantly influence breastfeeding duration and the maintenance of lactation.*
	Encourage mother to answer her other children's questions.
	Role play with mother possible situations related to questions of her child(ren).
Family sleep patterns are maintained with minimal disruption	Discuss sleep pattern disruptions that may occur.
	Encourage significant others to demonstrate their support by assisting with household responsibilities.
	Provide praise and positive reinforcement to family members.
Family trips are not curtailed	Discuss how to plan family trips that are conducive to breastfeeding.

References 17, 29, 158, 200, 316, 328, 419, 425, 505, 632.

Breastfeeding, Ineffective

Related factors: Previous history of breastfeeding failure; poor infant suck reflex

Michele C. Gattuso and Mi Ja Kim

PATIENT GOALS/ EXPECTED OUTCOMES	NURSING INTERVENTIONS/ SCIENTIFIC RATIONALE
Establish optimal lactation as evidenced by the following:	
Verbalizes accurate information related to breastfeeding	Review patient's knowledge of effective breastfeeding.
Identifies personal and family support for breastfeeding	Encourage patient/significant others to verbalize emotional attitudes about breastfeeding.
Able to feed infant with minimal assistance	Observe for presence of flat or inverted nipples.
Infant nurses at least every 3 hours	Use nipple shells. *The nipple protrudes through a hole in the center and constant gentle pressure around the nipple causes it to evert.*
Infant is satisfied between feedings	Demonstrate techniques to help infant "latch on" correctly. *Incorrect position of the infant's mouth abrades the nipple, causing soreness.*
	Observe infant during feeding for faulty sucking mechanism.
	Demonstrate colostrum expression to entice infant.
	Promote appropriate positioning for feeding: side-lying, football hold, sitting, or across abdomen.
	Provide for frequent feedings on demand every 2 to 3 hours around the clock.
	Do not restrict sucking time.
	Offer both breasts at each feeding; demonstrate burping between breasts.
	Provide suggestions for waking a sleepy baby.

continued.

BREASTFEEDING, INEFFECTIVE

PATIENT GOALS/ EXPECTED OUTCOMES	NURSING INTERVENTIONS/ *SCIENTIFIC RATIONALE*
Maintain the breastfeeding process as evidenced by the following:	
Mother expresses confidence in her ability to handle future situations Mother identifies resources for problems/support	Provide supplement only when medically indicated. *Substitute bottles may confuse infant.* Discourage delaying or skipping of feedings. Discuss and observe for signs of adequate let-down reflex. Provide for rest periods. Discuss breastfeeding diet, such as increased protein, calcium, and calories. Discuss implications for using medications while breastfeeding. *Passive diffusion causes passage of a drug from plasma to milk.* Demonstrate use of assistive devices for infants with poor suck reflex. Provide support and positive reinforcement. Identify resources and support groups for breastfeeding. Describe how mother can tell whether baby is getting enough milk (e.g., daily weights, level of irritability). Provide anticipatory guidance for developmental changes that affect breastfeeding (i.e., growth spurts). Discuss role of father/significant other while breastfeeding. Discuss effects of breastfeeding on sexuality.

Breastfeeding, Ineffective—cont'd

PATIENT GOALS/ EXPECTED OUTCOMES	NURSING INTERVENTIONS/ SCIENTIFIC RATIONALE
Mother has fewer breast complications as evidenced by the following:	
No evidence of breast/nipple trauma	Observe breast for engorgement, warmth, redness of nipple, cracks or fissures in nipple, or anomaly of breast.
Verbalizes minimal breast/nipple discomfort	Encourage frequent nursings with proper positioning.
Verbalizes/demonstrates breast care techniques	Apply warm, moist packs 10 to 15 minutes before feeding or encourage patient to take warm showers before feeding.
Verbalizes satisfaction with breastfeeding	Massage all around breast, moving from outer margin toward nipple.
	Hand express or pump breast to soften areola and make nipple protrude.
	Expose nipples to air dry after each feeding.
	Discourage use of soaps or lotions containing alcohol.
	Apply ointments as prescribed after each feeding.
	Encourage patient to begin feedings on least sore breast.
	Teach proper technique to break suction of nursing infant.
	Vary position of infant's mouth on breast by changing holding position with each feeding.
	Provide analgesics as prescribed.
	Encourage use of supportive bra 24 hours a day.
	Observe return demonstration of appropriate breast care techniques.

References 143, 316, 328, 403, 407, 498, 539.

Related factor: Prematurity

Emma B. Nemivant and Mi Ja Kim

PATIENT GOALS/ EXPECTED OUTCOMES	NURSING INTERVENTIONS/ SCIENTIFIC RATIONALE
Demonstrate a commitment to breastfeed the preterm infant as evidenced by the following:	
Participates in initial consultation with nurse with expertise in breastfeeding premature infants	Encourage mother to consult (NICU) breastfeeding specialist. *NICU breastfeeding specialist has expertise in both lactation and in the clinical care of high risk infants.* Provide privacy during consultation.
Recognizes the immunological, nutritional, and emotional benefits of breastfeeding as they relate to the infant's special condition	Reinforce the immunological and nutritional benefits of breastfeeding. *Milk produced by mothers who deliver preterm infants differs in composition from milk produced by mothers who deliver at term. Preterm milk has higher concentrations of protein, sodium, calcium, lipids, and selected antiinfective properties, which is consistent with the unique nutritional needs of preterm infants. Evidence indicates that breastfeeding affords protection against illness, generally, and respiratory and gastrointestinal infections, specifically, during infancy.* Discuss the emotional benefits of breastfeeding. *Mothers of preterm infants have stated repeatedly that breastfeeding is the one thing they can do for their preterm infants when professionals have assumed other caregiving activities.*

Breastfeeding, Interrupted—cont'd

PATIENT GOALS/ EXPECTED OUTCOMES	NURSING INTERVENTIONS/ SCIENTIFIC RATIONALE
Recognizes that the expressed milk will be given to the infant by artificial feeding method such as gavage	Provide information to the mother that most small, preterm infants cannot be breastfeed directly. Therefore they receive expressed mother's milk (EMM) by artificial feeding such as gavage infusion until they have demonstrated the ability to feed orally. *Preterm infant's ability to coordinate sucking, swallowing, and breathing varies from 32 to 36 weeks of gestation depending on feeding method.*
Perform correct milk expression and maintain adequate milk supply as evidenced by the following: Pumps breasts 8 to 12 times daily in the early postpartum period Uses recommended pump and collecting equipment for optimal production of milk Continues expression of milk per schedule for 2 weeks at home after infant's discharge	Develop a workable plan that incorporates physiological principles of early and frequent milk expression in the postpartum period. *Stimulating lactation is easier in the early postpartum period than it is several days later. Milk produced in early lactation, especially colostrum, contains antiinfective properties that are more beneficial to the infant. Frequent pumping contributes to adequate supply of milk.* Encourage the patient to rent an electric breast pump with a double pump collecting kit for use at home *to optimize prolactin levels and decrease pumping times.* Reinforce the importance of adequate nutrition, fluids, and rest *to ensure adequate milk supply.*

continued.

Breastfeeding, Interrupted—cont'd

PATIENT GOALS/ EXPECTED OUTCOMES	NURSING INTERVENTIONS/ *SCIENTIFIC RATIONALE*
	Discuss on individual basis concerns related to medications, smoking, or alcohol ingestion while mother is expressing milk for her preterm infant. *Depending on maternal dosage and clinical condition of the infant, drug that is considered "safe" if present in EMM for full-term healthy infants may not be equally safe for a 750-g, 26-week infant.*
	Teach mother the correct use of pump, proper cleaning, and the assembly and disassembly of equipment.
	Inform mother that with few exceptions, pumping will continue for at least 2 weeks after the infant has been discharged from NICU *to completely empty breasts and increase prolactin levels.*
	Help with breast pump rentals and purchases from referral agencies *so as to relieve mother of the burden of phone calls at a stressful time. Nurse's assistance ensures services from the agencies that benefit the mother, such as (1) the delivery of appropriate pump and collecting equipment, (2) direct billing of third-party payers, if the mother so desires, and (3) pick up of the pump from the mother's home when no longer needed.*

Breastfeeding, Interrupted—cont'd

PATIENT GOALS/ EXPECTED OUTCOMES	NURSING INTERVENTIONS/ *SCIENTIFIC RATIONALE*
Produce expressed mother's milk (EMM) with "abnormally" low bacteriological contamination as evidenced by the following:	
EMM has an absence of all bacteria except skin flora in minimal concentrations (e.g. 10^2 to 10^4 colony-forming units (cfu) per ml)	Develop protocol for maternal breast care and bacteriological surveillance of EMM. *EMM is never sterile and contains staph epidermidis that may be pathogenic to preterm infants.*
Willingly complies with the established protocol for milk expression	Teach mothers about bacteria-reducing techniques for milk expression as recommended by Meier and Wilks.[387] *The smaller, sicker preterm infant has a compromised immune system and may be more susceptible to bacteria in EMM.*
	Explain the milk expression techniques and the reasons for special precautions. *Assure mother that her hygiene is not being questioned but that the precautions are to reduce the bacteria to "abnormally" low levels.*
	Send mother's EMM for culture per protocol *to ensure that mother is exercising appropriate expression techniques.*

continued.

BREASTFEEDING, INTERRUPTED

PATIENT GOALS/ EXPECTED OUTCOMES	NURSING INTERVENTIONS/ SCIENTIFIC RATIONALE
Follow proper techniques for handling and storage of expressed mother's milk (EMM) as evidenced by the following:	
Uses recommended containers for storage of EMM to minimize the bacteriological contamination skin flora concentration at 10^2 to 10^4 colony-forming units (cfu) per ml Uses EMM within 24 hours after refrigeration	Instruct mothers to collect EMM in sterile, graduated plastic feeders with twist-on, air-tight caps that are easily handled by the nurses who will prepare the milk for gavage or bottle feeding. *Such feeders are ideal for EMM storage and easier to defrost and handle without contaminating the contents.* Label each bottle with baby's name, date, time milk was pumped, and any medication the mother is taking. Advise mother to use fresh and/ or previously frozen EMM for feeding within 24 hours after refrigeration. *No definitive guidelines are available for the length of time EMM can remain refrigerated until it is fed to the infant, except for conservative policy based on American Academy of Pediatrics Committee on Nutrition.* Encourage mother to express milk just before each feeding. *This approach is optimal in minimizing bacterial growth and maximizing antiinfective properties of the milk received by the infant.*

References 11a, 60, 262, 284, 316, 383, 385, 387, 420, 438, 625.

Breathing Pattern, Ineffective

Related factors: Respiratory muscle weakness and/or fatigue, impaired respiratory mechanics*
Janet L. Larson and Mi Ja Kim

PATIENT GOALS/ EXPECTED OUTCOMES	NURSING INTERVENTIONS/ *SCIENTIFIC RATIONALE*
Minimize energy expenditure of respiratory muscles as evidenced by the following:	
Respiratory rate slowed, tidal volume increased, and dyspnea decreased.	Teach pursed lip breathing, abdominal stabilization, and controlled coughing techniques; provide optimal care for mechanical assistance (e.g., ventilator) if necessary. *Pursed lip breathing forces patients to breathe more slowly and deeply and reduces dyspnea during exertion. Adbominal stabilization and controlled coughing techniques provide support to the expiratory muscles and assist in removing airway secretions while minimizing energy expenditure.*
Increase inspiratory muscle strength and endurance as evidenced by the following:	
Increases maximal inspiratory pressure and reports decreased exertional dyspnea	Evaluate status of inspiratory muscles for training and, if appropriate, initiate inspiratory muscle training. *Inspiratory muscle training improves conscious control of respiratory muscles and decreases anxiety associated with increased inspiratory effort. Increased strength of the inspiratory muscles may allow some patients to tolerate submaximal levels of activity for longer periods with less dyspnea.*

*For the patient with stable COPD.

continued.

BREATHING PATTERN, INEFFECTIVE

PATIENT GOALS/ EXPECTED OUTCOMES	NURSING INTERVENTIONS/ *SCIENTIFIC RATIONALE*
	Monitor oxygen saturation with pulse oximeter during training session to verify that patient does not desaturate. Encourage patient to breathe as deeply as possible during inspiratory muscle training. *Using very small tidal volumes during inspiratory muscle training could cause some patients to experience oxyhemoglobin desaturation.*
Limit work of breathing as evidenced by the following:	
Reports taking prn antibiotics when sputum color changes (yellow or green)	Teach patient to monitor color, consistency, and volume of sputum because respiratory infections increase work of breathing. *Early treatment of a bacterial infection of the lungs may speed recovery and thereby reduce the work of breathing.*
Reports taking methylxanthines and beta agonists as prescribed	Teach patient name, dosage, method of administration, schedule, and appropriate behavior if side effects occur, and consequences of improper use of medications. *Both methylxanthines and beta agonists produce brochodilation and therefore decrease airway resistance and work of breathing. Both medications also have potentially dangerous cardiac toxicities, and for some produce distressing neurological symptoms such as shakiness and irritability.*

Breathing Pattern, Ineffective—cont'd

PATIENT GOALS/ EXPECTED OUTCOMES	NURSING INTERVENTIONS/ SCIENTIFIC RATIONALE
	Evaluate patient's technique for taking inhaled medications. Recommend a spacer device for patients who have difficulty with timing during the procedure. *Under optimal conditions, no more than 10% of the drug from each puff is deposited into the lungs; with a spacer device, as much as 15% of the drug will be deposited.*
Demonstrates ability to pace ADLs in line with ventilatory function.	Teach patient to modify ADLs within ventilatory limits.
	Induce periodic hyperinflation of lungs with a series of slow, deep breaths. *Hyperinflation works like a deep sigh, expanding alveoli that are partially closed, mobilizing airway secretions and increasing lung tissue compliance.*

BREATHING PATTERN, INEFFECTIVE

PATIENT GOALS/ EXPECTED OUTCOMES	NURSING INTERVENTIONS/ *SCIENTIFIC RATIONALE*
Maintain normal respiratory rate, depth, and ratio of inspiratory and expiratory times as evidenced by the following: Rate, depth, and inspiratory-expiratory ratio of respirations remain within normal limits	Continue to monitor rate and depth of respiratory breath sounds, use of accessory muscles of respiration, and sensations of dyspnea. *Clinical manifestations of respiratory muscle fatigue include rapid shallow breathing in early stages with an increase in $Paco_2$ level and decrease in respiratory rate in the late stages. Accessory muscles of respiration will be employed as the work of breathing increases. Respiratory muscle fatigue magnifies sensations of dyspnea.* Continue to monitor ratio of inspiratory time/total duration of respiration. *An increase in the ratio of inspiratory time to total duration of respiration is less efficient for the inspiratory muscles.*

Breathing Pattern, Ineffective—cont'd

PATIENT GOALS/ EXPECTED OUTCOMES	NURSING INTERVENTIONS/ *SCIENTIFIC RATIONALE*
	Continue to observe for abnormal chest wall motion as an indication of increased inspiratory workload. This is manifested by paradoxic motion, which is characterized by expansion of the ribcage and inward motion of the abdomen during inspiration. Asynchronous chest wall motion is characterized by disorganized and uncoordinated respiratory motion.

References 15, 47, 290, 302, 315, 345, 410, 527, 581, 597.

Cardiac Output, Decreased

Related factors: Electrophysiological rhythm disturbance: bradyarrhythmias (heart rate <40/minute) or tachyarrhythmias (heart rate >180/minute)*

Margaret J. Stafford and Mi Ja Kim

PATIENT GOALS/ EXPECTED OUTCOMES	NURSING INTERVENTIONS/ *SCIENTIFIC RATIONALE*
Regain normal range of cardiac output (CO) as evidenced by the following: Normal blood pressure for patient Cardiac rate/rhythm within normal range, free of bradyarrhythmias and/or tachyarrhythmias without IV medication; with or without maintenance oral medications; with or without pacemaker therapy; with or without support of automatic internal cardioverter defibrillator (AICD) Absence of ST-T wave changes on ECG Expresses being free of chest pain/discomfort, dyspnea, dizziness, palpitations, and syncope **Experience less stress, fear, and anxiety as evidenced by the following:** Verbalizes understanding of and acceptance of therapy—drugs and treatment Relates positive social interaction	Assess/document/evaluate the patient's response to the bradyarrhythmias or tachyarrhythmias and signs/symptoms associated with decreased CO (e.g., altered mentation, dizziness, hypotension, pallor, diaphoresis, dyspnea, abnormal breath sounds or heart sounds, feelings of anxiety or alarm, fatigue, palpitations, chest pain, and loss of consciousness). Determine the need for continuous monitoring in collaboration with the physician. Explain, if indicated, the purpose of the ICU or surveillance unit to patient/significant others and reassuringly discuss the advantages of "having your heartbeat watched continuously."

*For the patient with acute myocardial infarction.

Cardiac Output, Decreased—cont'd

PATIENT GOALS/ EXPECTED OUTCOMES	NURSING INTERVENTIONS/ SCIENTIFIC RATIONALE
	Symptomatic bradyarrhythmia, heart rate ≤40 beats/minute Evaluate the patient's response to the slow rate and hemodynamic disorders. Bradycardia (<40 beats/minute) causes symptoms of decreased perfusion as CO is compromised due to the slow rate (CO = SV × HR). Review patient's current medications to identify drugs that could decrease the heart rate (e.g., morphine sulfate, a vagomimetic agent; verapamil, a calcium blocker; proprandol, a beta blocker; or digoxin, a cardiac glycoside with potential side effects of bradycardia and AV block). Discuss with the physician the feasibility of discontinuing or substituting these drugs. Provide adequate ventilation and administer oxygen as indicated. Give a single chest thump (if appropriate) and encourage deep coughing to stimulate cardiac activity and improve CO. If the patient has a syncopal episode, lower the patient's head and raise the legs to facilitate cerebral circulation. Notify the physician stat.

continued.

PATIENT GOALS/ EXPECTED OUTCOMES	NURSING INTERVENTIONS/ *SCIENTIFIC RATIONALE*
	Initiate an IV and administer/titrate drugs (according to hospital policy/protocol; e.g., a bolus of atropine sulfate, 0.5 to 1.0 mg). If rate does not increase, repeat 0.5 mg doses every 5 minutes up to maximum of 2.0 mg. *Atropine* is a parasympatholytic agent that blocks the action of the vagus nerve, increasing heart rate and enhancing atrioventricular (AV) conduction.* Monitor for side effects (e.g., urinary retention, headache, dizziness and dryness, abdominal distention and pain, photophobia/glaucoma, and ectopic ventricular beats). Give with caution because *excessive increases in rate may worsen existing myocardial ischemia;* isoproterenol HCL (Isuprel*) is a synthetic *sympathomimetic drug with potent inotropic and chronotropic properties.* It may be given as a temporary measure when hemodynamic problems persist and until a temporary pacemaker can be inserted. Prepare 1 mg of Isuprel to 500 ml of 5% dextrose in sterile water (2 μg/ml). Infuse 2 to 10 μg/min titrated according to heart rate and rhythm response. Assist with insertion of a transvenous, temporary pacemaker if indicated and reassuringly explain its purpose and the process to the patient. Temporary pacing

*For the patient with MI, Isuprel and atropine may cause an extension of the infarct; vagal stimulation actually may be beneficial to diminish ventricular vulnerability.

Cardiac Output, Decreased—cont'd

PATIENT GOALS/ EXPECTED OUTCOMES	NURSING INTERVENTIONS/ SCIENTIFIC RATIONALE
	is indicated for the patient with severe bradycardia but with a palpable pulse and for the patient who has high-grade heart block whose conducted beat (intrinsic or pacemaker generated) results in a palpable pulse. When symptoms persist, a permanent pacemaker is considered.
	If a permanent pacemaker is implanted, provide a comprehensive/holistic plan of care, including the following factors: Involve the patient/significant others in establishing preoperative/postoperative and long-term goals; explain purpose/function of the pacemaker being implanted (e.g., physiological, rate responsive, single or dual); provide a pacemaker-specific teaching booklet reviewing the concepts with the patient; reassure/explain benefits of pacing related to energy level and dispel misconceptions about restrictions such as sexual activity and non-contact sports, but review appropriate precautions; reassure patient about cosmetic appearance and self-image in general; introduce concept of ECG telephone transmissions and clinic visits. Counsel the patient when fears and concerns persist. Review all medications— purpose, side effects, diet, and activity restrictions, if indicated, and promote positive "upbeat" attitude/behavior.

continued.

CARDIAC OUTPUT, DECREASED

PATIENT GOALS/ EXPECTED OUTCOMES	NURSING INTERVENTIONS/ *SCIENTIFIC RATIONALE*
	Tachyarrhythmias ***Heart rate ≥180 beats/minute*** Analyze the rhythm for regularity and the morphology of the complexes. Determine the site of origin of the tachyarrhythmia in the conduction system (arterial, junctional, or ventricular). Heart rates >180 that originate above the ventricles—referred to as supraventricular tachycardias (SVT) are not imminently life-threatening but may seriously compromise CO. *The diastolic filling time is shortened, diminishing preload, stroke volume, and ultimately decreasing CO.* *(CO = SV × HR.)*

Cardiac Output, Decreased—cont'd

PATIENT GOALS/ EXPECTED OUTCOMES	NURSING INTERVENTIONS/ *SCIENTIFIC RATIONALE*
	Assess the following in presence of SVT ≥180 beats/minute.† (1) Assess the quality of peripheral pulses and detect pulse deficits. In arterial fibrillation (and other arterial rhythms that are extremely fast and/or uncoordinated) the arterial contribution to CO (the "atrial kick") is lost by as much as 30%. (2) Monitor blood pressure for hypotension and signs of decreased perfusion and auscultate for extra heart sounds, specifically S3. When the left ventricle is failing and non-compliant, the sudden deceleration of the filling wave produces an audible third sound. (3) Monitor and evaluate the 12-lead ECG for precipitous changes and signs of myocardial ischemia (e.g., depressed ST segments and T-wave changes). (4) Determine the presence of and evaluate chest pain/discomfort. *With sustained tachycardia, there is the potential for decreased cardiac perfusion (related to the shortened diastolic filling time), decreased oxygen to the myocardium, and increased workload.* (5) Monitor pulmonary status and adverse behavior changes for potential emboli as a *result of disorganized arterial activity.* (6) If the patient is being anticoagulated, monitor prothrombin levels,

†The following general assessment factors and interventions relate to all fast rate arrhythmias >180 beats/minute originating above the ventricles unless stated otherwise. *continued.*

PATIENT GOALS/ EXPECTED OUTCOMES	NURSING INTERVENTIONS/ SCIENTIFIC RATIONALE
	and if not, discuss with the physician (if appropriate) the feasibility of anticoagulation. Initiate oxygen delivery, an IV, and hemodynamic monitoring as indicated and ordered. Notify the physician of significant changes and needed orders; initiate Valsalva maneuver or carotid sinus stimulation if indicated (per protocol). *These actions increase parasympathetic (vagal) responses, producing a block in the AV node and reducing the ventricular rate.*
	Administer and titrate (per protocol) medication as ordered (e.g., verapamil, *which interrupts the reentrant circuit and increases the delay in the AV node;* propranolol, *to decrease automaticity and conduction velocity slowing the heart rate;* and/or digoxin, *to slow AV conduction, increasing degrees of heart block and slowing the ventricular rate).* Monitor and report untoward reactions.

Cardiac Output, Decreased—cont'd

PATIENT GOALS/ EXPECTED OUTCOMES	NURSING INTERVENTIONS/ *SCIENTIFIC RATIONALE*
	Prepare the patient for electrical cardioversion if indicated and ordered. *Cardioversion delivers a synchronized direct current charge to the myocardium, causing all the cells to depolarize simultaneously and allowing the sinus node to gain control. Assist as indicated with synchronizing the "charge" with the patient's QRS to avoid the vulnerable period of the cardiac cycle and potential ventricular fibrillation.* Explain the procedure in accurate but nonthreatening terms, secure a written consent, and reassure the patient that he/she will receive a medication before the treatment to avoid pain and discomfort. If overdrive pacing is ordered, explain the treatment to the patient, secure a consent and assist as indicated. *Overdrive pacing is usually effective in controlling the fast rate and may convert some SVTs to normal sinus rhythm.* *Ventricular tachycardia (VT) not only causes a decrease in CO as described with SVTs, but also may rapidly progress to ventricular fibrillation and death.*

continued.

CARDIAC OUTPUT, DECREASED

PATIENT GOALS/ EXPECTED OUTCOMES	NURSING INTERVENTIONS/ *SCIENTIFIC RATIONALE*
	Assess level of consciousness and peripheral pulses. If the patient is unresponsive, not breathing, and pulseless, initiate CPR and alert the CPR team. If a defibrillator is immediately available, administer unsychronized counter shock stat at 200 watts and proceed with CPR as outlined in hospital policy.
	If the patient is conscious and hemodynamically stable, give a chest thump and instruct the patient to cough, *in an attempt to maintain consciousness.* Thump chest only if a back-up defibrillator is available, because doing so could precipitate ventricular fibrillation. Initiate drug regimen according to hospital policy (e.g., a 50- to 75-mg lidocaine bolus, followed by an IV infusion with lidocaine).
	Prepare the patient for overdrive pacing if indicated. Talk with the patient throughout the procedures, calmly and reassuringly explaining the treatment.
	Explain, before discharge, dosage and side effects of maintenance drugs (e.g., procainamide, quinidine, calcium channel blockers, beta blockers, and others as prescribed); discuss restrictions related to exercise, diet, modified lifestyle, and the need for follow-up care.

Cardiac Output, Decreased—cont'd

PATIENT GOALS/ EXPECTED OUTCOMES	NURSING INTERVENTIONS/ *SCIENTIFIC RATIONALE*
	If an AICD is implanted, a detailed teaching plan with the patient and family should include purpose, restrictions, how it works, what to do when it doesn't, CPR, and specific appointments for follow-up care.

References: 68, 99, 103, 115, 156, 188, 475, 552, 553.

Caregiver Role Strain

Related factors: Physical/emotional demands of caregiving role; perceived isolation of caregiver

Audrey M. McLane

PATIENT GOALS/ EXPECTED OUTCOMES	NURSING INTERVENTIONS/ *SCIENTIFIC RATIONALE*
Obtain assistance with meeting demands of caregiving role as evidenced by the following:	
	Identify caregiver resources and requirements for care.
Verbalizes caregiving tasks that could be delegated	Develop options for delegation of specific tasks within budgetary limits.
Obtains information about costs of home health-care services and respite care	Provide/discuss information about respite care. Provide caregiver with list of medical and financial resources in area.
Contracts with health-care providers for specific services	Help patient/caregiver develop a daily schedule that includes pacing direct care activities. *Delegation of specific task to formal caregivers may enable patient to remain in home setting despite an expected negative trajectory.*
Develop support system with friends and neighbors as evidenced by the following:	
Identifies social resources that could be mobilized	Help caregiver to identify type/ source of support that would be most helpful.
Requests that neighbor sit with patient while caregiver goes to church	Help caregiver to negotiate with patient to resume one preferred leisure time activity.
Invites a friend to come for tea and conversation once a week	

Caregiver Role Strain—cont'd

PATIENT GOALS/ EXPECTED OUTCOMES	NURSING INTERVENTIONS/ SCIENTIFIC RATIONALE
Maintain/improve care-giver's health status as evidenced by the following: Develops and implements a plan for daily exercise Makes and keeps appointments for annual physical/pelvic examinations	Develop a plan for monitoring caregiver's health status. Teach/monitor use of daily log for recording caregiver's activities, rest periods, and hours of sleep at night. Help patient/caregiver to develop an alternate plan for patient's care in the event of caregiver's illness. *Demands/stress of caregiving increase vulnerability by depleting energy reserves.*

References 62, 81, 82, 194, 201, 332, 631.

Risk factors: Competing role demands; illness severity of care receiver; caregiver health impairment*

Audrey M. McLane

PATIENT GOALS/ EXPECTED OUTCOMES	NURSING INTERVENTIONS/ *SCIENTIFIC RATIONALE*
Establish a pattern of care-giving that is compatible with role demands as evidenced by the following:	
Negotiates with employer for temporary reduction in work hours without loss of benefits Requests alternating weekend assistance from daughter and son who live within driving distance	Formulate with caregiver alternatives for decreasing role demands (e.g., temporary reduction in work hours; use of formal health care services, such as respite care). Provide caregiver with a list of home health-care providers and financial resources in the community. *Early recognition of "at risk" status by caregiver will facilitate realistic planning for discharge.*
Provide competent care for recipient as evidenced by the following:	
Requests information/assistance with complex care activities Makes/keeps appointments to participate in patient care activities before discharge Verbalizes confidence in ability to provide care Contracts with health-care providers for specific services	Help patient/caregiver to develop a written plan of care. Determine caregiver's competence to carry out required care. Provide instruction/demonstration of patient care activities. Discuss with caregiver importance of spending time with patient when no care is being provided. *Patient needs to feel the nurturing aspects of the relationship in contrast to "burden" of care.*

*Caregiver is employed full time and is the primary wage earner.

Caregiver Role Strain, High Risk for—cont'd

PATIENT GOALS/ EXPECTED OUTCOMES	NURSING INTERVENTIONS/ *SCIENTIFIC RATIONALE*
Establish a self-care pattern consistent with role demands and caregiver's health impairment as evidenced by the following:	
Uses guest bedroom to sleep at night	Negotiate with patient/caregiver for separate sleeping arrangement with some form of communication.
Equips guest bedroom with electronic monitor to respond to patient's needs during night	Teach caregiver/recipient how to recognize signs/symptoms of fatigue.
Maintains nutrition adequate to maintain optimal health status	Teach importance of keeping light levels low during night to prevent difficulty in falling asleep after responding to patient's request for assistance.
	Provide caregiver with information about high energy food *to maintain optimal health status.*

References 62, 81, 82, 194, 201, 332, 631.

Communication: Impaired Verbal

Related factors: Psychological barriers

Gertrude K. McFarland and Charlotte E. Naschinski

PATIENT GOALS/ EXPECTED OUTCOMES	NURSING INTERVENTIONS/ *SCIENTIFIC RATIONALE*
Transmit clear, concise, and understandable messages as evidenced by:	
Selects and organizes words appropriate to receiver and context	Use facilitative communication techniques when interacting with patient.
Uses effective communication techniques	Teach and support use of effective communication techniques.
Uses appropriate amount of verbiage	Teach and support use of assertive communication skills.
Expresses feelings appropriately	Encourage initiation of conversations.
	Encourage expression of feelings.
	Use of effective communication techniques—such as reflection, validation, and clarification—results in transmission of understandable messages.
Attend to appropriate stimuli, as evidenced by the following:	
Selects and responds to relevant stimuli	Reduce stimuli to assist patient in attending to appropriate stimuli or increase stimuli to motivate patient.
Perceives stimuli accurately	Give clear, simple messages using language patient can understand.
Demonstrates orientation to time, place, and person	Teach patient to identify and focus on relevant stimuli.
	Assist in correction of faulty perception.

Communication: Impaired Verbal—cont'd

PATIENT GOALS/ EXPECTED OUTCOMES	NURSING INTERVENTIONS/ *SCIENTIFIC RATIONALE*
	Through manipulation of the environment, teaching, and role modeling, the nurse facilitates the patient's accurate perception of and response to stimuli.
Use congruent verbal and nonverbal communication as evidenced by the following:	
Demonstrates congruent verbal and nonverbal communication	Match verbal and nonverbal communication during nurse-patient interactions. Validate meaning of nonverbal communication.
Shows congruent nonverbal behaviors	Point out discrepancies in verbal and nonverbal communication.
Balances use of verbal and nonverbal communication	Point out discrepancies in message sent and context within which it is sent. Teach and encourage use of stress reduction techniques. *The message component of communication depends on translation of ideas, purpose, and intent into congruent verbal and nonverbal communication.*

continued.

Communication: Impaired Verbal—cont'd

PATIENT GOALS/ EXPECTED OUTCOMES	NURSING INTERVENTIONS/ SCIENTIFIC RATIONALE
Send and receive feedback as evidenced by the following:	
Listens actively	Encourage interaction with others.
Examines effects of behavior on others	Help patient develop understanding of dynamics of relationships.
Asks for and receives feedback	
Sends feedback to others	Increase patient's awareness of strengths and limitations in communication with others.
Uses feedback in the communication process	Describe, demonstrate, and encourage use of active listening skills.
	Provide feedback to patient.
	Teach patient to request feedback when communicating with others.
	Help patient to accept and send both positive and negative feedback.
	Support efforts to use feedback.
	Communication is modified or corrected through the regulatory process of feedback.
Experience gratification from communication as evidenced by the following:	
Sends and receives confirmation when communicating	Provide confirming responses to patient.
Reports or shows willingness to assume responsibility for communication	Teach and support use of confirming responses when communicating with others.
Reports satisfaction from communication	Teach patient evaluation of own and others' communication.
	Demonstrate and support responsibility for communication.

Communication: Impaired Verbal—cont'd

PATIENT GOALS/ EXPECTED OUTCOMES	NURSING INTERVENTIONS/ *SCIENTIFIC RATIONALE*
	Motivation to communicate is related to the gratification experienced from communication.

References 132, 193, 369, 370, 418, 509.

Constipation

CONSTIPATION

Related factors: Inadequate fluid and fiber in diet; daily
ingestion of constipating medications
Audrey M. McLane and Ruth E. McShane

PATIENT GOALS/ EXPECTED OUTCOMES	NURSING INTERVENTIONS/ *SCIENTIFIC RATIONALE*
Experience fewer incidences of constipation as evidenced by the following:	
Obtains immediate relief	Use lubricated, gloved finger to break up large masses of hard stool. Follow with tap-water enema or insert Dulcolax suppository within 1 hour of breakfast to *take advantage of gastrocolic reflex.*
	Exclude fatty acids from breakfast or triggering meal. *Fatty acids delay reflex stimulation and slow digestion.*
Takes fiber supplement once a day	Recommend use of fiber supplement once a day while on constipating medications with increase to twice a day if needed
Reports return to usual pattern of elimination: every 1-2 days	
Verbalizes understanding of constipating effects of selected medications	Teach patient about constipating effects of medications such as codeine.
Increase ingestion of fluids and fiber-rich foods as evidenced by the following:	
Eats bran muffin or bread daily	Teach patient to record all intake for 48 hours.
	Analyze eating pattern with patient.
	Recommend diet changes to increase bulk in diet.
Eats one high-fiber vegetable daily	
Verbalizes increase in fluid intake to 8-10 glasses daily	Recommend intake of 8 glasses of water daily.

References 376, 377, 378, 379, 380.

Constipation, Colonic

Related factors: Restricted mobility requiring use of equipment or device; preference for nonfibrous foods.

Audrey M. McLane and Ruth E. McShane

PATIENT GOALS/ EXPECTED OUTCOMES	NURSING INTERVENTIONS/ SCIENTIFIC RATIONALE
Establish a regular pattern of bowel movements as evidenced by the following:	
Has bowel movement at least every 3 days	Suggest trial of Dulcolax suppository instead of oral laxatives within 1 hour of breakfast or triggering meal, *which will elicit gastrocolic reflexes. Reflexes are strongest when the stomach is empty.*
Stool passes easily	
Experiences sensation of complete passage of stool	
Responds immediately to urge to defecate	Establish toileting routine.
	Teach patient/family importance of immediate response to urge to defecate. *Stool will harden in rectum in the presence of chronic distention.*
Modify dietary intake to change ratio of low-/high-fiber foods as evidenced by the following:	
Eats bran in some form daily	Teach patient and caregivers to record all intake for 48 hours.
Eats one high-fiber vegetable daily	Analyze eating pattern with patient and caregivers.
Substitutes whole grain for white bread	Recommend diet changes to increase bulk in diet, consistent with financial limitations.
	Recommend gradual addition of dietary fiber; 6 to 10 g of fiber each day. *Slow addition of fiber helps to avoid cramping and flatus.*

continued.

PATIENT GOALS/ EXPECTED OUTCOMES	NURSING INTERVENTIONS/ *SCIENTIFIC RATIONALE*
Increase activity level as evidenced by the following:	
Walks independently with cane or walker	Encourage outdoor walking (weather permitting).
Increases length of walks 10 ft per week	Increase ambulation distance from 20 ft to 40 ft and then to tolerance level.
Active range of motion (ROM) three times a day	Teach active ROM. *Inadequate exercise is a major contributor to change in stool consistency.*
Exercises abdominal muscles three times a day	Teach abdominal strengthening exercises.

References 377, 378, 379, 380, 466.

Constipation, Perceived

Related factors: Cultural/family health beliefs (expect to have daily bowel movement); overuse of laxatives.
Audrey M. McLane and Ruth E. McShane

PATIENT GOALS/ EXPECTED OUTCOMES	NURSING INTERVENTIONS/ *SCIENTIFIC RATIONALE*
Modify cultural family health beliefs with respect to need for daily bowel movement as evidenced by the following:	
Verbalizes acceptance of bowel movement every 2 to 3 days	Explore and acknowledge health beliefs and convictions. Confront health beliefs that maintain dysfunctional behaviors. *Out-of-date information leads to faulty appraisal of pattern of elimination and need for laxatives.*
Modify toileting routines as evidenced by the following:	
Drinks hot liquid before breakfast	Prescribe lemon juice and hot water every morning for 1-week trial. Teach patient to recognize and attend to stimulus behaviors (i.e., actions/behaviors that stimulate urge to defecate). *Gastrocolic reflexes are strongest when stomach is empty.*
Reports use of rectal suppository less than once a week	Teach patient use of suppository to stimulate evacuation.

continued.

Constipation, Perceived—cont'd

CONSTIPATION, PERCEIVED

PATIENT GOALS/ EXPECTED OUTCOMES	NURSING INTERVENTIONS/ *SCIENTIFIC RATIONALE*
Decrease use of laxatives as evidenced by the following: Substitutes fresh fruit and vegetable sticks for candy or desserts in lunches	Provide instruction about use of bulk and fiber in brown-bag lunches. Discuss temporary use of Metamucil to supplement natural fiber in diet.
Gradually increases walking to 1 mile, 4 times a week	Teach patient role of exercise in developing and maintaining acceptable pattern of bowel elimination.

References 377, 378, 379, 380.

Coping, Defensive

Related factors: Stressful event; threat to self-esteem*
Linda O'Brien-Pallas, Margaret I. Fitch, and Gertrude K. McFarland

PATIENT GOALS/ EXPECTED OUTCOMES	NURSING INTERVENTIONS/ *SCIENTIFIC RATIONALE*
Experience defenses that are protected against threat as evidenced by the following:	
No suffering from further insult to self-esteem	Support patient's personhood, uniqueness, and right to be involved in decision making.
	Seek to understand patient's perspective of situation and what is stressful or threatening. Specifically, seek to understand patient's sense of self and role expectations of self. *Enhancing an individual's self-esteem involves, as a first step, exploring the discrepancies within his/her self-concept.*
	Encourage maintenance of social support.
	Assist patient in becoming aware of behaviors that are harmful to others (e.g., ridicule), but do not try to move patient from defensive stance.
Move away from use of defensive behaviors as evidenced by the following:	
Verbalizes a realistic appraisal of the event, its demands, and coping resources available	Assist patient in exploring nature and characteristics of breast cancer's demands and coping resources required: identify where discrepancies exist between ideal and perceived roles in the situation. *Pace intervention to patient's readiness for assistance because a period of denial may be present.*
Verbalizes comfort with ideal and perceived roles and competencies to manage situation	
Communicates a sense of personal integrity	

*For the patient with diagnosis of carcinoma of the breast. *continued.*

COPING, DEFENSIVE

PATIENT GOALS/ EXPECTED OUTCOMES	NURSING INTERVENTIONS/ *SCIENTIFIC RATIONALE*
	Help patient to identify desired goals.
	Where possible, reduce stressful aspects of the event and enhance patient's coping abilities through: setting realistic, concrete goals with individual; identifying specific strategies for achieving goals; setting realistic timeframes for reaching goals; reviewing capabilities and learning from past experiences; exploring patterns of thinking (especially negative thoughts); teaching necessary knowledge and skills; acknowledging accomplishments toward desired goals; maintaining social networks; and encouraging expression of fears and concerns. *Pacing interventions with the patient's progression helps the patient adapt to the situation.*

References 5, 131, 247, 318, 319.

Coping, Family: Potential for Growth

Contextual factors: Adaptive tasks effectively addressed;
progress toward self-actualization
Martha M. Morris and Gertrude K. McFarland

PATIENT GOALS/ EXPECTED OUTCOMES	NURSING INTERVENTIONS/ *SCIENTIFIC RATIONALE*
Actualize growth potential of a crisis as evidenced by the following:	
Verbalizes changes in family roles/relationships	Identify changes in family dynamics resulting from crisis.
Verbalizes changes in individual attitudes, values, and goals	Identify changes in individual family members resulting from crisis.
Chooses goals and experiences that foster growth and achieve self-actualization	Discuss goals and experiences that maximize growth potential.
	Provide information as needed to enable individuals/family to develop new goals that relate to individuals and total family system and methods of achieving such goals.
	Facilitate development of new methods of goal attainment and self-actualization.
	Most families may be viewed as healthy, but in need of temporary support. Interventions aimed at promoting family competence provide temporary support.
Develop broader base of support as evidenced by the following:	
Verbalizes interest in contacting others experiencing a similar situation	Identify patient/family readiness to accept support from additional sources.
Contacts additional persons/groups when referred	Refer patient/family to appropriate resources.
Develops additional relationships that provide support during crisis	Initiate contact if necessary.

continued.

Coping, Family: Potential for Growth—cont'd

PATIENT GOALS/ EXPECTED OUTCOMES	NURSING INTERVENTIONS/ *SCIENTIFIC RATIONALE*
Sustains contact with additional sources	Follow up to ensure sustained contact and appropriateness of assistance. *Individual/family should be aided in developing a broader base of support, which will maximize growth potential.*

References: 63, 98, 265, 323, 334.

Coping, Ineffective Family: Compromised

Related factors: Inadequate understanding by family member (father); temporary family disorganization*
Martha M. Morris and Gertrude K. McFarland

PATIENT GOALS/ EXPECTED OUTCOMES	NURSING INTERVENTIONS/ *SCIENTIFIC RATIONALE*
Experience increasing comfort as evidenced by the following:	
Displays decreased levels of anxiety as environment is perceived as supportive	Maintain as much privacy as possible.
Verbalizes feelings to healthcare professionals and other family members	Provide alternative to patient's room for family discussion.
	Provide information about hospital routines, services, and facilities.
	Encourage family member to verbalize feelings such as loss, guilt, or anger.
	Use communication techniques that confirm legitimacy of both positive and negative feelings (e.g., reflecting feelings ["You seem frightened"], presenting reality ["Many people feel angry during this situation"]).
Develop adequate understanding of situation as evidenced by the following:	
Verbalizes need for more information or clearer understanding relating to breast cancer and related treatment	Provide adequate and correct information to patient and family member.
Demonstrates understanding of information given	Discuss "sick role" with patient and family member.
Discusses changes in mother and her family as result of mother's illness	Encourage family to have realistic perspectives based on accurate information.
	Discuss usual reactions to major health challenges, such as anxiety, dependency, and depression.

*For the family with mother recently diagnosed and hospitalized with breast cancer.   *continued.*

PATIENT GOALS/ EXPECTED OUTCOMES	NURSING INTERVENTIONS/ SCIENTIFIC RATIONALE
	Provide opportunities for patient to discuss need for support with family member.
	Monitor areas in which knowledge or understanding is inadequate in relation to a major illness.
	Encourage patient and family members to discuss expectations with each other.
	Supportive and informational family education is essential in helping a family that is coping ineffectively.
	Fostering a sense of "family" within an educational climate can promote family growth.
Cope with changes in family processes as evidenced by the following:	
Identifies changes in family processes as a result of the mother's illness	Help family to appraise the situation, including family's strengths and weaknesses.
Recognizes roles needed to maintain family integrity	Help family to identify changes in relationships as a result of mother's illness.
Assumes new roles as necessary to maintain family integrity	Help family member to recognize role changes needed to maintain family integrity.
Family member (father) participates in care of mother	Involve family member in care of patient as much as possible.
	Refer family member to appropriate additional sources for help in adjusting to changes in family processes.
	Restructuring of role relationships can increase family competence.

Coping, Ineffective Family: Compromised—cont'd

PATIENT GOALS/ EXPECTED OUTCOMES	NURSING INTERVENTIONS/ *SCIENTIFIC RATIONALE*
	Encouragement to use sources outside the family may be appropriate to preserve the supportive capacity of family members in assuming new roles over time.

References 63, 226, 291, 323, 324.

Coping, Ineffective Family: Disabling

COPING, INEFFECTIVE FAMILY: DISABLING

Related factors: Dissonant discrepancy of coping styles; highly ambivalent family relationships

Gertrude K. McFarland and Martha M. Morris

PATIENT GOALS/ EXPECTED OUTCOMES	NURSING INTERVENTIONS/ *SCIENTIFIC RATIONALE*
Achieve accurate understanding of conflicts in coping styles as evidenced by the following:	
Verbalizes perception(s) of coping styles and areas of conflict	Help family members and patient to verbalize own perceptions of coping styles and areas of conflict.
Identifies alternative coping behaviors that may minimize conflict	Help family members and patient to identify alternative coping behaviors to minimize conflict in adapting to health challenge.
	Identify areas of conflict in coping styles among individuals within family unit.
	Monitor individual and family coping styles.
Develop alternate coping strategies as evidenced by the following:	
Uses effective coping strategies	Help family members and patient to focus on present feelings.
Incorporates alternate coping behaviors in adapting to health challenge	Assist family members and patient in practicing alternative coping behaviors (e.g., relabeling, role playing, contracting). *A family with limited understanding about various coping strategies may need information about alternatives, as well as the potential effect of conflict of coping styles. To incorporate new behaviors, the patient and family member may require assistance in learning alternative coping behavior.*

Coping, Ineffective Family: Disabling—cont'd

PATIENT GOALS/ EXPECTED OUTCOMES	NURSING INTERVENTIONS/ *SCIENTIFIC RATIONALE*
Achieve improved level of complementarity in role relationships as evidenced by the following:	
Discusses complementary nature of strengths, needs, and expectations of relationships	Help patient and family members to verbalize individual needs and expectations of relationships during present health challenge.
Identifies areas in which needs and expectations are not being met	Help patient and family members to identify individual strengths and weaknesses in adapting to health challenge.
	Assist patient and family members to discuss areas where individual strengths, needs, and expectations complement each other in adapting to health challenge.
	Help patient and family members to identify needs and expectations that are not being met.
Identifies strategies to aid developing complementary relationships	Help patient and family members identify additional strategies to develop complementary relationships in adapting to health challenge.
Incorporates alternative strategies in relationships	Assist patient and family members in practicing new strategies.
	A family experiencing disabling anxiety as a result of inability to cope with the changes in role relationships imposed by a health challenge may be assisted by helping them to identify the changes that have occurred.

continued.

Coping, Ineffective Family: Disabling—cont'd

COPING, INEFFECTIVE FAMILY: DISABLING

PATIENT GOALS/ EXPECTED OUTCOMES	NURSING INTERVENTIONS/ *SCIENTIFIC RATIONALE*
	Once needs and expectations have been explored, specific strategies to develop complementary relationships in the current situation can be identified and practiced.

References 19, 219, 299, 366, 614.

Coping, Ineffective Individual

Related factors: Inadequate response repertoire*
Evelyn L. Wasli and Gertrude K. McFarland

PATIENT GOALS/ EXPECTED OUTCOMES	NURSING INTERVENTIONS/ SCIENTIFIC RATIONALE
Develop an adequate response repertoire as evidenced by the following: Verbalizes or demonstrates the cognitive knowledge learned, the skill achieved, and the new behavior acquired Uses the new knowledge, behavior, and skill in daily life activities	Assist patient in identifying the need he/she wishes to meet or the goal he/she wants to achieve *to enhance engagement in the coping process.* Support acknowledgment of feelings, wants, desires, fears, "bad habits," and impulses that need control. Discuss the consequences of feelings of rejection, social isolation, and other thoughts and feelings. Assist in seeking ways to turn thoughts and feelings into a motivational force for patient in achieving goals or meeting needs. Identify the basic response repertoire needed (e.g., stress management; health management; coping skills such as basic living skills, communication, assertiveness, leisure management, problem solving, leadership, and cognitive functioning; educational and occupational training; and maintaining social support.

*For the patient with undifferentiated schizophrenia.

continued.

COPING, INEFFECTIVE INDIVIDUAL

PATIENT GOALS/ EXPECTED OUTCOMES	NURSING INTERVENTIONS/ *SCIENTIFIC RATIONALE*
	Provide or refer the patient for the appropriate learning (e.g., for patient with undifferentiated schizophrenia who experiences a deficit in social skills, provide social skills training).
	Monitor deficits in social skills as specifically as possible (i.e., lack of assertiveness, poor eye contact, expressionless responses, inappropriate voice tone, inability to converse with others, difficulty with everyday interactions, lack of problem-solving skills, or attention impairments).
	In collaboration with patient, specify interpersonal problems patient has had in social interaction (e.g., communication skills).
	Have patient role play an interpersonal situation.
	Assess patient's receiving skills (e.g., What cues are being attended to? Are various aspects of the situation perceived? Is there an awareness of the relationship aspects of the interaction?)
	Identify collaboratively with patient new behaviors to be learned.
	Engage patient in role playing problem interactions.

Coping, Ineffective Individual—cont'd

PATIENT GOALS/ EXPECTED OUTCOMES	NURSING INTERVENTIONS/ *SCIENTIFIC RATIONALE*
	Use a variety of techniques to modify each component of behavior (i.e., facial expression, voice content). Give positive feedback as patient learns new skills or behavior. Designate specific tasks to be completed in real-life setting and give feedback about progress. Evalute progress in developing social skills to cope with crises at regular intervals.

References 74, 89, 121, 208, 330, 350, 464, 456, 596.

Decisional Conflict (About Seeking Prenatal Genetic Counseling and Testing)

Related factors: Unclear goals and values; unrealistic expectations

Annette M. O'Connor and Gertrude K. McFarland

PATIENT GOALS/ EXPECTED OUTCOMES	NURSING INTERVENTIONS/ SCIENTIFIC RATIONALE
Make and implement an informed choice that is consistent with personal goals and values as evidenced by the following:	
Understands what genetic counseling and testing can achieve	Explore patient's goals and clarify alternatives and their possible consequences. *Lack of information or clarity of these items contributes to decisional conflict.*
Expresses realistic consequences of having and not having prenatal testing Values the consequences as positive and negative	Realign unrealistic expectations. *Distortion in expectations often increases conflict (e.g., anticipating a negative consequence when the likelihood is extremely low) or regret (e.g., anticipating a positive consequence when the likelihood is extremely low).*
Identifies priority of anticipated consequences and implicit tradeoffs in the selection process	With the patient, clarify the desirability of possible consequences and their priority. *Unclear values contribute to decisional conflict.* Identify value tradeoffs implicit in making choices. *Having to make tradeoffs often contributes to conflict. Knowing what makes the decision difficult helps in its resolution.*
Selects course of action consistent with personal values	Facilitate alternative selection consistent with personal values. *Value congruence increases satisfaction with the decision and the likelihood that the patient will follow through on the choice.*

Decisional Conflict (About Seeking Prenatal Genetic Counseling and Testing)–cont'd

PATIENT GOALS/ EXPECTED OUTCOMES	NURSING INTERVENTIONS/ *SCIENTIFIC RATIONALE*
Uses self-help skills in implementing selected course of action Expresses satisfaction with the decision made	Teach and reinforce self-help skills required to implement the choice. *Individuals have difficulty implementing decisions made without the resources necessary to do so.*

References 273, 287, 450, 504, 540, 541.

DENIAL, INEFFECTIVE

Related factor: Life-threatening event*
Linda O'Brien-Pallas, Jane E. Graydon, and Gertrude K. McFarland

PATIENT GOALS/ EXPECTED OUTCOMES	NURSING INTERVENTIONS/ SCIENTIFIC RATIONALE
Maintain appropriate level of denial as evidenced by the following:	
Remains appropriately defended	Focus on establishing a trust relationship with patient.
	Determine patient's degree of denial and effectiveness of same as a coping strategy *because some degree of denial may be necessary for patient functioning.*
	If patient is using full denial, make periodic checks as to patient's stage of denial.
	Support patient's behavior.
	Never directly confront patient's denial *because the patient may not be able to handle the resulting anxiety.*
Acknowledges some degree of problems and concerns	Provide patient with specific information and/or reassurance if he/she should raise any questions or concerns.
	Do not push patient to raise questions or concerns if he/she is not ready. *Working with the patient in terms of his/her particular stage of denial at any point in time is important.*

References 72, 180, 224, 318, 531, 576, 613.
*For the patient with myocardial infarction (MI).

Diarrhea

Related factors: Careless food preparation and preservation; infrequent handwashing
Audrey M. McLane and Ruth E. McShane

PATIENT GOALS/ EXPECTED OUTCOMES	NURSING INTERVENTIONS/ SCIENTIFIC RATIONALE
Establish a normal pattern of bowel movements as evidenced by the following:	
Decreases number of stools to less than 3 per day Stools are formed Free of abdominal pain	Obtain stool for culture and sensitivity if diarrhea continues. Evaluate medication profile for gastrointestinal side effects. Teach patient appropriate use of antidiarrheal medications. *Antidiarrheal drugs are not recommended for routine use in acute infectious diarrhea, because they may delay the natural eradication of the infection.* Instruct patient/family members to record color, volume, frequency, and consistency of stools. *Volume of diarrheal fluid is an important indicator of the mechanism of the diarrhea. High volume (>1 L/day) suggests small intestinal origin. Small volume suggests colonic origin.*
Gain weight as evidenced by the following:	
Increases body weight 1 lb per week	Refer patient for consultation with a physician if diarrhea persists and is accompanied by weight loss. Teach patient/spouse how to keep a food diary for 48 hours. Evaluate recorded intake for nutritional content. Encourage frequent, small feedings (add bulk gradually).

continued.

Diarrhea—cont'd

PATIENT GOALS/ EXPECTED OUTCOMES	NURSING INTERVENTIONS/ SCIENTIFIC RATIONALE
Monitor/improve health practices to identify factors contributing to diarrhea as evidenced by the following:	
Eliminates irritating foods from diet	Teach patient to eliminate gas-forming and spicy foods from diet.
Eliminates lactose and other suggested food items from diet	Suggest trial elimination of foods containing lactose.
Makes and keeps medical appointments	
Practices good handwashing techniques	Teach/monitor improved handwashing.
Develops improved practices for food preparation and preservation	Demonstrate/monitor safe food preparation/preservation.

References 106, 378, 484, 605.

Disuse Syndrome, High Risk for

Risk factor: Immobilization

Maureen E. Shekleton and Mi Ja Kim

PATIENT GOALS/ EXPECTED OUTCOMES	NURSING INTERVENTIONS/ SCIENTIFIC RATIONALE
Maintain joint movement, muscle size and strength, and bone mineralization as evidenced by:	
Full ROM in joints	Perform active/passive ROM exercises *to maintain functional integrity of muscles and joints through use, prevent disuse atrophy of muscles, and prevent contracture development in muscles and joints through stretching of connective tissue.*
Muscle size and strength within normal limits	Perform isometric muscle setting exercises *to maintain muscle tone.*
	Maintain anatomic positioning of limbs *to maintain structural integrity of muscles and joints and prevent contracture development.*
	Dangle at bedside as tolerated.
	Assist patient up to chair as tolerated.
Ability to bear weight without discomfort.	Ambulate as tolerated. *Weight bearing prevents calcium loss through increased bone deposition.*

continued.

PATIENT GOALS/ EXPECTED OUTCOMES	NURSING INTERVENTIONS/ *SCIENTIFIC RATIONALE*
Maintain adequate systemic and local tissue perfusion as evidenced by the following:	
Blood pressure remains normal and no complaint of dizziness during position changes	Perform bed exercises as tolerated *to promote venous return and CV work capacity.*
Peripheral pulses remain intact	Apply antiembolism stockings *to prevent venous pooling in extremities.*
No dependent edema formation	
No complaint of weakness/fatigue with activity	Perform positional change in relation to gravity as tolerated: supine, semi-upright, and upright *to prevent decreased orthostatic capacity by enhancing neurovascular tone.*
	Actively contract muscles of lower extremities when assuming upright position *to increase muscle pumping of pooled blood to increase venous return and maintain cardiac output.*
Promote feelings of independence and control as evidenced by the following:	
Does not verbalize feelings of powerlessness or loss of control	Allow opportunity for decision making regarding care *to increase patient's sense of control related to situation and environment.*
Participates in self-care and ADLs to maximal extent possible	Encourage participation in ADLs as tolerated.
Patient and family/significant others express satisfaction with patient's progress and treatment	Encourage independence in self-care activities.
	Introduce and encourage use of assistive devices prn.

Disuse Syndrome, High Risk for—cont'd

PATIENT GOALS/ EXPECTED OUTCOMES	NURSING INTERVENTIONS/ *SCIENTIFIC RATIONALE*
Maintain normal skin and tissue integrity as evidenced by the following:	
Skin remains dry, pink, warm, and intact, especially over bony prominences and pressure points	Reposition at least every 1 to 2 hours *to relieve pressure and promote tissue perfusion.*
Maintains normal tissue turgor, elasticity, and strength	Encourage adequate intake of fluid and diet *to provide tissue hydration and nutrient supply.*
	Provide adequate protein in diet *to maintain positive nitrogen balance.*
	Inspect all pressure points at least every 2 hours.
	Provide clean, dry, and wrinkle-free bedding.
	Use assistive pressure-relief devices as needed (e.g., foam mattress, gel flotation pads, air-fluidized bed).
Maintain normal patterns of elimination as evidenced by the following:	
Urine output within normal limits	Encourage adequate fluid intake *to increase volume of urine and water volume of stool.*
Urine remains clear, light yellow, and without sediment	Get patient up to bathroom or commode as tolerated. *Anatomic position will facilitate complete emptying of bladder and bowel aided by gravity and muscle contraction.*
Urine specific gravity is 1.010-1.025	
Bowel movement per regular pattern	
Stool soft and formed	Provide adequate roughage (fiber, fruit, vegetables) in diet as tolerated *to provide bulk and stimulate peristalsis.*
Absence of discomfort when urinating or defecating	Provide acid-ash diet *to maintain acidity (lower pH level) of urine.*
	Give stool softener/laxatives as indicated.

continued.

PATIENT GOALS/ EXPECTED OUTCOMES	NURSING INTERVENTIONS/ *SCIENTIFIC RATIONALE*
	Provide privacy during act of voiding/defecation.
Maintain appropriate and adequate sensory stimuli as evidenced by the following:	
Remains oriented to time, person, and place	Provide access to clock, radio, television, and reading materials.
	Encourage visits from others.
	Maintain normal day/night light patterns.
	Avoid monotonous sensory stimuli.
Maintain effective breathing pattern and patent airway as evidenced by the following:	
Expectorates secretions	Perform deep breathing and coughing exercises every hour *to promote respiratory muscle excursion and mobilize secretions.*
Breath sounds clear	
Tidal volume, negative inspiratory force (NIF), and vital capacity within normal limits	
Chest excursion is complete and equal bilaterally	Encourage adequate fluid intake *to provide hydration to keep secretions loose and moist.*
	Monitor breath sounds.

References 221, 309, 326, 442, 529, 583.

Diversional Activity Deficit

Related factors: Limited leisure resources; long-term hospitalization*
Gertrude K. McFarland and Karen E. Inaba

PATIENT GOALS/ EXPECTED OUTCOMES	NURSING INTERVENTIONS/ *SCIENTIFIC RATIONALE*
Identify strengths and limitations in engaging in diversional activities as evidenced by the following:	
Sets realistic goals for diversional activities	Review patient's usual pattern of diversional activities *to assess activity level, tolerance, and preferences.*
Seeks out realistic opportunities for involvement in diversional activities	Assist patient in describing desired or required activity level changes because of altered health status.
Adapts diversional activities to changing health status	Assist patient in discussing limitations in usual pattern of diversional activities *to provide information about perceived and actual stressors that influence activity level.*
	Provide opportunities to continue meaningful diversional activities that are realistic within current environment *to support patient's sense of self-worth and productivity.*
	Include patient in making decisions about varying the daily routine *to promote a sense of control and recognition of personal preferences.*
	Facilitate opportunities for visits from friends and family *to stimulate social interaction and contact with the outside world.*

*For a geriatric patient in a long-term care facility who is confined after a total hip replacement.

continued.

Diversional Activity Deficit—cont'd

PATIENT GOALS/ EXPECTED OUTCOMES	NURSING INTERVENTIONS/ *SCIENTIFIC RATIONALE*
Identify strategies for obtaining needed resources as evidenced by the following: Assumes responsibility for choice of diversional activity Expresses acceptance of available diversional activity resources in current environment	Assist patient in identifying realistic resources and energy expenditures required to participate in meaningful activities. *Discussion provides opportunities for mutual goal setting and problem solving.* Inform patient about options for diversional activities available in setting (e.g., recreational therapy, occupational therapy, art/music therapy, remotivation therapy) *to assist in structuring free time and decreasing boredom.* Support patient's perceptions of resources needed for satisfying diversional activity requirements in individual situation (e.g., confinement).
Engage in satisfactory diversional activities as evidenced by the following: Expresses satisfaction with diversional activities Initiates and maintains participation in diversional activities available in current environment	Help patient assess any changes in ability to engage in preferred diversional activities. Adapt daily routine and use environmental structuring whenever possible to provide physical and mental stimulation and variety (e.g., change of scenery, creative activities) *to enhance socialization and involvement in the milieu.*

Diversional Activity Deficit—cont'd

PATIENT GOALS/ EXPECTED OUTCOMES	NURSING INTERVENTIONS/ SCIENTIFIC RATIONALE
	Encourage patient to verbalize about his/her own experience *to provide support and acknowledgement and to evaluate satisfaction with choice of activities.*
	Provide feedback to patient about level of participation in activities and observed self-structuring of free time. *Social reinforcement encourages continued efforts by the patient.*

References 1, 144, 186, 248, 268, 276, 469, 486, 506.

Dysreflexia

DYSREFLEXIA

Related factors: Distended bladder; cutaneous stimuli below T7*

Catherine Ryan and Mi Ja Kim

PATIENT GOALS/ EXPECTED OUTCOMES	NURSING INTERVENTIONS/ SCIENTIFIC RATIONALE
Prevent episodes of dysreflexia as evidenced by the following:	
Recognizes signs and symptoms of autonomic dysreflexia	Teach signs and symptoms of dysreflexia (e.g., elevation of blood pressure >20 mm Hg above patient baseline, pounding headache, bradycardia, sweating, piloerection, and facial flushing).
Demonstrates understanding of the effect of bladder distention to dysreflexia	Teach patient/significant others about methods to prevent bladder distention (e.g., Foley care, intermittent catheterization). *Bladder distention is the most common cause of autonomic dysreflexia.*
	Maintain adequate fluid intake. *Adequate fluid intake will help to prevent bladder infection.*
	Adhere to bowel training program. *Bowel distention may stimulate an episode of autonomic dysreflexia.*

*For the patient with spinal cord injury (T7 or above) who is at risk for recurrent episodes of autonomic dysreflexia.

Dysreflexia—cont'd

PATIENT GOALS/ EXPECTED OUTCOMES	NURSING INTERVENTIONS/ *SCIENTIFIC RATIONALE*
Recover from episode of dysreflexia without residual effects as evidenced by the following: Blood pressure and pulse within normal limits for patient Skin dry and without red splotches above the level of the lesion Absence of pallor below lesion	Remove stimuli for dysreflexia: examine urinary drainage system for obstruction; eliminate obstruction or remove catheter. Avoid performing Crede's maneuver. Catheterize if on intermittent catheter program. Assess for signs and symptoms of urinary tract infection. Loosen tight clothing or restrictive appliances. Apply topical anesthetic around anus and in rectum and check for/ manually remove fecal impaction. Inspect skin for evidence of pressure sore or rashes. *Sympathetic stimulation below T7 can stimulate an exaggerated, unopposed autonomic nervous system response. The response is exaggerated because the response cannot cross the injured area of the cord and is therefore unopposed by the parasympathetic nervous system.* Elevate head of the bed or place patient in sitting position. *Elevation of the head will create orthostatic hypotension and lower the blood pressure.* Monitor the blood pressure and pulse every 5 minutes during acute episode.

References 174, 372.

Related factor: Situational transition*

Evelyn L. Wasli and Gertrude K. McFarland

PATIENT GOALS/ EXPECTED OUTCOMES	NURSING INTERVENTIONS/ SCIENTIFIC RATIONALE
Family will achieve stabilized functioning as evidenced by the following: Views problem as having meaning for members of family unit, not just "the patient." Demonstrates constructive interaction of the family unit. Demonstrates problem solving from the identification of the problem to the evaluation of the action taken. Demonstrates appropriate role functioning in the family unit. Demonstrates affective responsiveness in the family unit. Demonstrates ability to set standards of behavior for the family unit.	Help family redefine situation in terms that lead to increased options and possibilities for change (not labeling of "patient," "bad," or faulting another system). *Redefinition assists family to reexamine the situation as a response to multiple stressors (e.g., new culture, loss of extended family, need to find new job, adjustment to illness—rather than blaming wife for refusing to adjust to the new situation).* Support efforts of family to clarify the who, what, when, where, and how of the stress and to identify their responses as a family unit. Assist family in problem solving by providing information, raising questions, assisting to summarize progress, and so on. Assist family in reallocating important functions during crisis period. *Setting priorities helps family use available energies to deal with most important family activities.*

*For a recently married couple immigrating to United States from Mexico. Wife recently diagnosed with anorexia nervosa.

Family Processes, Altered—cont'd

PATIENT GOALS/ EXPECTED OUTCOMES	NURSING INTERVENTIONS/ SCIENTIFIC RATIONALE
	Assist family in tolerating conflict, change, and expressions of stress in behavior of individual family members and in expressing appropriate concern and support to each other.
	Assist family to be flexible in setting and altering standards of behavior in times of stress (not that of "anything goes" or "do nothing" or "tell no one").

References 164, 205, 239, 304, 401.

Fatigue

FATIGUE

Related factors: Role demands; increased metabolic demands*
Sarah Anne Badalamenti, Patricia A. Koller, and Audrey M. McLane

PATIENT GOALS/ EXPECTED OUTCOMES	NURSING INTERVENTIONS/ *SCIENTIFIC RATIONALE*
Establish a pattern of rest/ activity that enables fulfill- ment of role demands as ev- idenced by the following:	
Negotiates realistic role expecta- tions	Help patient to identify exces- sive demands of various role obligations.
	Instruct patient to maintain a fa- tigue diary for a 1-week pe- riod.
Exercises 2 to 3 times a week within own tolerance	Monitor level of fatigue using Rhoden Fatigue Scale and the
Engages in preferred leisure 2-3 times a week	Fatigue Severity Scale. *Analy- sis of the relationship between*
Verbalizes decreased sense of fatigue	*activities and levels of fatigue will help define areas in which to reduce role demands and energy losses.*
	Formulate with patient options for decreasing work demands (e.g., reduction in work hours, delegation of selected tasks).
	Help patient to plan a daily schedule that includes pacing leisure activities, rest, and ex- ercise.
Verbalizes feeling well-rested on arising	Monitor sleep pattern.
	Teach patient to eliminate/re- duce physical activities 1 hour before bedtime. *A function of sleep is to restore both mental and physical energy.*

*For the patient who has lung cancer; is a business executive.

Fatigue—cont'd

PATIENT GOALS/ EXPECTED OUTCOMES	NURSING INTERVENTIONS/ *SCIENTIFIC RATIONALE*
Improve nutritional status as evidenced by the following: Stabilizes body weight Consumes well-balanced, high caloric diet based on individual needs	Teach use of food diary to monitor eating habits. Review food diary/food preferences. Help patient to identify foods high in protein and complex carbohydrates. Provide information on use of high-calorie food supplements. Teach patient/significant other short-cuts to meal planning/preparation. *Role demands and coping with the effects of illness increase energy demand and requirement for nutrients.*
Restore mental energy as evidenced by the following: Uses a relaxation technique at least once a day Verbalizes an increased sense of control.	Teach/monitor relaxation techniques agreeable to patient (i.e., progressive muscle relaxation, creative imagery, and music). Negotiate use of meditation or prayer. *Stress depletes energy, which contributes to fatigue. Relaxation techniques can be effective in stress management.*

References 6, 52, 213, 236, 301, 398, 416, 468, 599.

Related factors: Impending surgery with possible pain, loss of control, disfigurement*

Gertrude K. McFarland and Victoria L. Mock

PATIENT GOALS/ EXPECTED OUTCOMES	NURSING INTERVENTIONS/ *SCIENTIFIC RATIONALE*
Identify specific aspects of impending surgery that are sources of fear as evidenced by the following:	
Verbalizes specific fears relating to surgery, realistic perception of danger, own coping ability, and need for assistance	Using techniques of therapeutic communication, encourage patient to verbalize subjective feelings experienced, personal perception of danger, perception of own coping skills/limitations, and need for assistance from nursing staff. *Verbalizing feelings can lessen the intensity and duration of fear.*
Acquire knowledge/skills for dealing with specific fears as evidenced by the following:	
	Deal with distorted perceptions. Provide information to reduce distortions. Encourage specifics rather than generalizations. *A realistic appraisal promotes effective problem solving to decrease the danger.* Initiate teaching about surgery, including colostomy.
Verbalizes and displays comfort with unit environment, procedure, and staff	For unfamiliar environment, orient patient to unit and staff.
Comfortably demonstrates coughing, deep breathing, and leg exercises	Teach rationale and procedure for turning, coughing, deep breathing, and leg exercises; allow time for practice and return demonstration.

*For the patient with bowel cancer.

Fear—cont'd

PATIENT GOALS/ EXPECTED OUTCOMES	NURSING INTERVENTIONS/ SCIENTIFIC RATIONALE
	Knowledge of what to expect— particularly on a sensory level—decreases fear of the unknown.
Explains events expected to occur before and after surgery	Teach specifics for type of surgery.
Verbalizes realistic expectations for postoperative period	Teach what to expect after surgery (e.g., colostomy, irrigation, recovery wound dressings).
	Identify and teach specifics of the surgical experience that the patient would like to know.
	Avoid surprises: tell patient what to expect, especially sensations that will be experienced.
	For fear of pain, teach about postoperative analgesia.
	For fear of loss of control, teach ways of enhancing control (e.g., include patient in planning care; share test results as appropriate).
	For fear of disfigurement, consider visit by someone who has successfully experienced and is well adjusted to the surgery (e.g., colostomy). *Fear decreases when one identifies with someone who has successfully dealt with a similar fearful situation.*

continued.

PATIENT GOALS/ EXPECTED OUTCOMES	NURSING INTERVENTIONS/ *SCIENTIFIC RATIONALE*
Engage in adaptive coping as evidenced by the following:	
Verbalizes increased psychological comfort and coping skills	Use available support system to increase comfort and relaxation.
	Include family and significant others in teaching *so that they are supportive and knowledgeable, rather than fearful.*
	Encourage comforting measures (e.g., music, religious objects, own pajamas, pillow). *Familiar sources of comfort can alleviate the distress that accompanies fear.*
	Arrange a visit with clergy, if desired by patient
Verbalizes positive attitude toward outcome of surgery	Adopt a positive attitude that patient can cope and have a positive surgical experience
Experiences a restful sleep	Facilitate a good night's sleep preoperatively
Experience reduced fear as evidenced by the following:	
Verbalizes decreased fear	Continually monitor level of fear (many surgeons will cancel surgery if patient is especially fearful). *The neuroendocrine physiological response to fear may precipitate life-threatening arrhythmias during stressful situations.*
Pulse and respiration rates normal	

References 100, 212, 235, 408, 436, 571.

Fluid Volume Deficit (1)

Related factor: Failure of regulatory mechanism*
Kathryn Czurylo and Mi Ja Kim

PATIENT GOALS/ EXPECTED OUTCOMES	NURSING INTERVENTIONS/ *SCIENTIFIC RATIONALE*
Maintain adequate fluid volume and electrolyte balance as evidenced by the following:	
Afebrile and blood pressure and pulse within normal limits for patient	Monitor vital signs every 15 minutes until stable.
Glucose under 300 mg/dl	Administer insulin per order according to blood glucose levels: *Insulin is required to reverse hyperglycemia.*
	Maintain IV therapy for replacement of fluid per order.
	Administer replacement K^+ therapy for hypokalemia as appropriate. *Osmotic diuresis causes K^+ depletion; also, insulin administration causes K^+ to shift intracellularly.*
Intake and output balanced Stable weight	Monitor intake and output every hour and weigh patient daily *because these provide a good measure of body fluid balance.*
Urine specific gravity within normal limits (1.010-1.025)	Monitor specific gravity of urine every 2 hours.
	Monitor urine electrolytes and report abnormal values.
Hct/Hgb levels within normal limits Electrolytes within normal limits Serum osmolarity level within normal limits	Monitor serum electrolytes (especially Na^+ and K^+), Hct/ Hgb, and serum osmolarity values and report abnormal values.
	Monitor for circulatory overload during fluid replacement (e.g., neck vein distention, rales, dyspnea, S-3, increase in CVP or PAP, and tachycardia).

*For the patient with hyperglycemic hyperosmotic nonketotic coma (HHNC).

continued.

Fluid Volume Deficit (1)–cont'd

FLUID VOLUME DEFICIT (1)

PATIENT GOALS/ EXPECTED OUTCOMES	NURSING INTERVENTIONS/ *SCIENTIFIC RATIONALE*
	Continue to monitor and report to physician worsening fluid volume deficit/electrolyte imbalance signs and symptoms (e.g., dilute urine, increased urine output, hypotension, increased pulse rate, decreased skin turgor, increased body temperature, and weakness). Monitor level of consciousness.

References 214, 217, 241, 327, 341, 342, 457.

Fluid Volume Deficit (2)

Related factors: Active loss of body fluid*
Kathryn Czurylo and Mi Ja Kim

PATIENT GOALS/ EXPECTED OUTCOMES	NURSING INTERVENTIONS/ *SCIENTIFIC RATIONALE*
Maintain adequate fluid volume and electrolyte balance as evidenced by the following:	
Blood pressure and pulse within normal limits for patient	Determine cause of active loss and use nursing actions to prevent further loss. Monitor vital signs every hour.
Skin turgor within normal limits	Monitor skin condition: color, moisture, turgor. Maintain IV therapy for replacement of fluid using colloids, crystalloids, or blood products per order. *Colloids hydrate the intravascular space and pull fluids from the interstitium into the blood stream; crystalloids replace extracellular fluid and are distributed to the interstitium and intravascular space; and blood replacement must be given to provide oxygen-carrying capacity if hemoglobin is significantly decreased.* Push PO fluids to 2600 ml/day if appropriate.
Intake and output balanced	Monitor intake and output every hour and report urine output of less than 30-60 ml/hour. *Urine volume decreases in hypovolemia, because decreased plasma volume results in decreased renal blood flow.*
Stable weight	Weigh patient at the same time daily. *Weights with intake and output provide a good measure to body fluid balance.*

*For the patient with hypovolemic shock. *continued.*

PATIENT GOALS/ EXPECTED OUTCOMES	NURSING INTERVENTIONS/ *SCIENTIFIC RATIONALE*
Urine specific gravity within normal limits (1.010-1.025)	Monitor urine specific gravity every 2 hours; *concentrated urine (specific gravity >1.030) is response to water deficit as ADH is released in response to increased osmolarity of body fluids.*
Electrolyte levels within normal limits	Monitor serum electrolytes Monitor for circulatory overload during fluid replacement (e.g., neck vein distention, rales, dyspnea, S-3, increase in CVP or PAP, and tachycardia). Monitor and report worsening fluid volume deficit and/or electrolyte imbalance signs and symptoms (e.g., decreased urine output, concentrated urine, output greater than intake, hypotension, increased pulse rate, increased body temperature, weakness, and change in mental status). Monitor level of consciousness.

References 217, 259, 341, 393, 457, 546.

Fluid Volume Deficit, High Risk for

Risk factor: Daily use of diuretics*
Kathryn Czurylo and Mi Ja Kim

PATIENT GOALS/ EXPECTED OUTCOMES	NURSING INTERVENTIONS/ SCIENTIFIC RATIONALE
Maintain adequate fluid volume and electrolyte balance as evidenced by the following:	
Patient/family verbalizes knowledge of monitoring fluid status	Teach patient/significant other the following:
Serum electrolyte levels within normal limits	Daily weights and intake and output record keeping *because these provide a good measure of body fluid balance.*
Weight within normal limits for patient	Record blood pressure.
No excessive thirst	Importance of maintaining regular schedule of taking diuretics and K^+ supplements and eating K^+-rich foods, such as bananas, oranges, and raisins; *thiazide diuretics may result in potassium depletion.*
	Action and side effects of diuretics as necessary.
	Importance of good nutrition and fluid intake *because adequate fluid intake is important to prevent dehydration.*
	Change positions slowly *to minimize orthostatic hypotension.*
	Monitor skin turgor and avoid excessive dryness. *Poor skin turgor and dryness may indicate dehydration.*
	Avoid excessively hot environments *because heat may cause excessive water loss.*

*For the cardiac patient taking diuretics for congestive heart failure and/or hypertension.
References 20, 313, 457.

Fluid Volume Excess

FLUID VOLUME EXCESS

Related factor: Impaired myocardial contractility
Mi Ja Kim and Margaret J. Stafford

PATIENT GOALS/ EXPECTED OUTCOMES	NURSING INTERVENTIONS/ *SCIENTIFIC RATIONALE*
Achieve normal level of fluid volume as evidenced by the following:	
	Administer diuretics as ordered; teach patient the rationale for this medication. *Lasix is an effective and fast acting "loop" diuretic blocking Na^+ and Cl^- transport in the ascending limb. It produces less electrolyte loss than other diuretics. It increases the effective circulating to normal/acceptable range blood volume, thus decreasing preload.*
Body weight is within patient's normal range	Weigh patient daily and consult physician to adjust diuretic dosage as necessary.
Hemodynamic status is restored to normal/acceptable range without medication	
Electrolyte level stays within normal range	Monitor serum level of electrolytes, particularly K^+. *If hypokalemia develops, a flat or inverted T wave or a prominent U wave may appear.* The nurse may need to provide a K^+-rich diet with appropriate patient teaching and consult physician for K^+ supplement as necessary.
	Restrict fluid intake in presence of dilutional hyponatremia with serum Na^+ level below 130 mEq/L and monitor intake and output daily; *excessive water intake will cause further dilution of Na^+ in the blood.*

Fluid Volume Excess—cont'd

PATIENT GOALS/ EXPECTED OUTCOMES	NURSING INTERVENTIONS/ *SCIENTIFIC RATIONALE*
	Provide reduced Na^+ diet (range 1.2 to 1.6 g daily, if indicated) and teach patient that high Na^+ level induces fluid retention. Eliminate table salt and offer herbs/spices as an alternative to salt. Administer and teach about inotropic agents, such as digitalis, if necessary and ordered. *Inotropic agents will increase myocardial contractility.* Explain and titrate vasopressor agents (e.g., dopamine, dobutamine) and/or vasodilator agent (e.g., sodium nitroprusside, hydralazine) if ordered. *Dopamine at low dosages (1 to 2 μ/kg/min) increases renal blood flow, promoting diuresis. Dobutamine produces positive inotropic effect and decreases preload. Sodium nitroprusside has a dual action, dilating both arterioles and veins, with a dramatic decrease in preload and afterload.* Monitor for toxic side effects of drugs.

Fluid Volume Excess—cont'd

PATIENT GOALS/ EXPECTED OUTCOMES	NURSING INTERVENTIONS/ *SCIENTIFIC RATIONALE*
	Monitor hemodynamic status by reading mean arterial pressure (MAP) and pulse pressure (via arterial line if available). *MAP indicates overall perfusion pressure of tissues/organs. Pulse pressure provides an estimate of the heart's stroke volume or pumping ability and is an index of the resistance to left ventricular emptying (afterload); central venous pressure (CVP) detects hemodynamic changes in the right side of the heart; pulmonary artery pressure (PAP) and pulmonary capillary wedge pressure (PCWP) secure an accurate evaluation of the volume of blood in the left ventricle before contraction (preload); cardiac output (CO) (indirect determination via the Swan-Ganz) indicates a response to therapy.* Consult physician if values exceed acceptable ranges.
	Monitor laboratory results relevant to fluid retention (e.g., increased specific gravity; presence of protein, urea, and granular casts in urine; increased BUN; increased mean corpuscle volume (MCV); and decreased hematocrit).

Fluid Volume Excess—cont'd

PATIENT GOALS/ EXPECTED OUTCOMES	NURSING INTERVENTIONS/ SCIENTIFIC RATIONALE
Experience less discomfort due to excessive fluid volume as evidenced by the following:	
Verbalizes less dyspnea and experiences more comfort	Provide position that will allow fluid shift and help alleviate dyspnea (e.g., semi-Fowler's position).
	Provide support to edematous areas (e.g., pillow under arms and scrotal support).
	Teach passive and active ROM exercises if appropriate.
	Provide high-protein and high-calorie diet *to enhance the healing of the waterlogged body tissue,* if present.
	Counsel patient if significant changes in sensorium exist or concerns are expressed about body image and self-esteem as a result of excessive fluid retention.
	Provide appropriate skin care if edematous and monitor potential for infection.

References 23, 116, 190, 222, 394, 471, 475, 517, 522, 582.

GAS EXCHANGE, IMPAIRED

Related factors: Altered oxygen supply; alveolar hypoventilation

Mary V. Hanley and Mi Ja Kim

PATIENT GOALS/ EXPECTED OUTCOMES	NURSING INTERVENTIONS/ *SCIENTIFIC RATIONALE*
Maintain adequate oxygen supply and alveolar ventilation as evidenced by the following:	
Hypoxemia is resolved or improved with or without oxygen supplement or mechanical ventilation	Maintain patent airway while patient is both awake and asleep.
Performs techniques that maximize ventilation and perfusion matching	Encourage patient to take deep breaths (see Airway Clearance, Ineffective, p. 79).
Eucapnia or usual compensated Paco$_2$ and pH levels	Position patient to facilitate ventilation/perfusion matching ("good side down"). *Positioning affects distribution of pulmonary circulation and ventilation. Position patient so that most normal area of lung is dependent.*
	Remove secretions by coughing or suctioning (see Airway Clearance, Ineffective, p. 79).
	Consult physician about supplementary oxygen during activity and/or sleep. If ordered, select devices that enable the patient to perform ADLs and teach patient accordingly.
	Counsel patient who has chronic hypoxemia to obtain supplementary oxygen prescription from physician before air travel or trips to high altitude.
	If hypoxemia persists, consult physician for possible mechanical assistance or ventilation.

Gas Exchange, Impaired—cont'd

PATIENT GOALS/ EXPECTED OUTCOMES	NURSING INTERVENTIONS/ *SCIENTIFIC RATIONALE*
	If mechanical ventilation is prescribed, monitor ventilator settings, endotracheal and tracheal tube function, and function of ventilator and breathing circuits. Assess patient's ability to wean daily. Initiate weaning and support oxygenation requirements as described above. *Weaning is the titration of the intervention of mechanical ventilation. A patient's ability to wean depends on a number of physiological and psychological varibles (e.g., control of breathing, respiratory muscle strength and endurance, lung mechanics, gas exchange, as well as the patient's psychological readiness to be separated from the ventilator).*
	If mechanical ventilation becomes long-term, assess for home management by self or significant other (see Ventilation, Inability to Sustain Spontaneous, p. 350).
Impairment of mental status and restlessness are absent or reduced	Monitor mental state, including restlessness, coherency, and state of alertness.

References 12, 13, 15, 152, 202, 249, 300, 427, 434, 585, 593, 594, 617.

GRIEVING, ANTICIPATORY

Related factor: Perceived potential loss of spouse*
Gertrude K. McFarland and Elizabeth Kelchner Gerety

PATIENT GOALS/ EXPECTED OUTCOMES	NURSING INTERVENTIONS/ SCIENTIFIC RATIONALE
Wife participates in constructive anticipatory grief work as evidenced by the following:	
Discusses thoughts and feelings related to potential loss of spouse	Encourage wife to describe perceptions of potential loss *to identify specific aspect of grieving process wife is experiencing.*
	Encourage verbalization of fears, concerns, and other emotions. *The patient's verbalizations of anger are not personal attacks, and they facilitate the grieving process.*
Uses appropriate resources (e.g., friends, clergy, support groups, legal consultants, Social Security representative, and mental health professionals)	Determine current sources of social support, such as family, friends, and church and disruptions in current life-style related to potential loss of spouse, such as finances, living arrangements, and transportation. *Social support is an important resource to assist patient/wife during this health crisis.*
	Evaluate need for referral to resources, such as mental health professional for wife and/or children, referral to school counselor for children, Social Security representative, legal consultant, or grief support groups.
	Provide assurance that experiencing intense, chaotic feelings and reactions is normal *to minimize wife's concerns that she is experiencing abnormal reactions.*

*For the wife of spouse with nonHodgkin's lymphoma and graft versus host rejection.

Grieving, Anticipatory—cont'd

PATIENT GOALS/ EXPECTED OUTCOMES	NURSING INTERVENTIONS/ *SCIENTIFIC RATIONALE*
	Avoid judgmental and defensive responses to criticisms of health care providers. *Careful evaluation of criticism is essential to differentiate between valid criticism and criticism generated as a result of displaced anger related to potential loss of spouse.*
Meets ongoing self-care needs	Encourage wife to maintain her own self-care needs for rest, sleep, nutrition, leisure activities, and time away from patient *for her to maintain her own health and also continue to provide support to spouse.*
	Discuss indicators of change in physical condition of husband as appropriate.
	Provide wife with ongoing information of patient's diagnosis, prognosis, progress, and plan of care *to help her constructively engage in anticipatory grieving.*
	Encourage wife to describe desires and information needs in caring for patient.
	Facilitate wife's assistance with patient's physical care.
	Enlist support from others, such as family, friends, and clergy.
	Facilitate flexible visiting hours and include younger children when appropriate.
	Help wife and spouse to share mutual fears, concerns, plans, and hopes with each other.
Maintains constructive family functioning as a unit	Provide comforting measures for husband; encourage wife and significant others to assist if they wish.

continued.

GRIEVING, ANTICIPATORY

PATIENT GOALS/ EXPECTED OUTCOMES	NURSING INTERVENTIONS/ *SCIENTIFIC RATIONALE*
	Demonstrate competence by meeting husband's psychosocial and physical needs promptly and with empathy.
	Encourage wife and significant others to maintain verbal communication and touch with their loved one during times that patient may not be able to respond.
	Provide as much privacy as possible for wife and others to be alone with patient *for them to share freely.*

References 8, 120, 135, 155, 230, 481, 482, 503, 569, 615.

Grieving, Dysfunctional

Related factors: Loss of health; death of spouse*
Gertrude K. McFarland and Elizabeth Kelchner Gerety

PATIENT GOALS/ EXPECTED OUTCOMES	NURSING INTERVENTIONS/ *SCIENTIFIC RATIONALE*
Experience absence of de-layed emotional reactions as evidenced by the following: Acknowledges awareness of losses Verbalizes thoughts and feelings related to death of spouse and loss of health.	Monitor patient's current level and pattern of mood, energy, appetite, elimination, and vital signs *to determine response to treatment for hyperthyroidism and to differentiate from signs and symptoms of dysfunctional grieving.* Monitor patient's perception of current adaptation to loss of spouse and loss of health and degree of pattern of use of coping skills/problem-solving abilities and available social support. *These interventions support strengths, reinforce adaptive coping skills, and foster patient self-reliance. Perception of social support is a positive indicator for resolution of grieving.* Differentiate between helpful and maladaptive use of denial *to avoid unnecessary confrontation and to avoid reinforcement of maladaptive denial.* Observe for responses by health-care providers that may be reinforcing maladaptive denial of the patient. Point out reality in a non-threatening manner without arguing with patient or significant others.

*For the elderly widow experiencing multiple losses—hyperthyroidism and loss of spouse.

continued.

GRIEVING, DYSFUNCTIONAL

PATIENT GOALS/ EXPECTED OUTCOMES	NURSING INTERVENTIONS/ *SCIENTIFIC RATIONALE*
	Gradually present patient with more significant facts *to facilitate awareness of losses and to lay groundwork for adaptive behaviors.*
	Clarify and offer missing factual information.
	Facilitate constructive working through feelings by demonstrating tolerance for expression of negative feelings, supporting verbalizations of ambivalence, facilitating contact with persons who can openly express feelings, and helping patient to understand possible reasons for feelings. *Working through intense feelings facilitates resolution of grief and allows for engagement in problem solving.*
	Point out universality of need for normal grieving.
	Encourage description of recovery expectations and goals.
	Offer realistic hope for positive coping in the present, as well as the future.
Experience resolution of dysfunctional grieving as evidenced by the following:	
Follows prescribed treatment for hyperthyroidism	Encourage description of current and anticipated problems related to loss of health and loss of spouse.
Develops goals that are congruent with individual values and beliefs	Promote patient's recognition of past and present strengths that can be used for coping with current loss.
Identifies alternate plans for meeting goals that were significant before loss of spouse	

Grieving, Dysfunctional—cont'd

PATIENT GOALS/ EXPECTED OUTCOMES	NURSING INTERVENTIONS/ *SCIENTIFIC RATIONALE*
	Promote description of various strategies for coping with losses.
	Assist patient to develop realistic goals and life-style changes.
	Evaluate need for referral to resources, such as brief psychotherapy, support and spiritual counseling.
	Provide guidance about available community resources.
	Facilitating, encouraging, and teaching patient about use of own health team, family, and community resources will assist patient's adjustment to changes resulting from experience of overlapping losses.
	Facilitate contact with others who have successfully adapted to a similar loss.
	Encourage family and friends to offer support by visiting patient frequently on a regular basis.

References 189, 244, 317, 397, 447, 467, 497, 557, 560, 633.

Growth and Development, Altered

GROWTH AND DEVELOPMENT, ALTERED

Related factors: Inadequate maternal caretaking; environmental and stimulation deficiencies*

Carol Kupperberg and Gertrude K. McFarland

PATIENT GOALS/ EXPECTED OUTCOMES	NURSING INTERVENTIONS/ SCIENTIFIC RATIONALE
Reach maximal potential in mental and physical development as evidenced by the following: Meets physical and emotional needs	Monitor child's cognitive, social and psychomotor development. Monitor height and weight at regular intervals. *Diagnosis of fetal alcohol syndrome (FAS) requires manifestations in 3 categories: (1) prenatal or postnatal growth retardation (below tenth percentile for gestational age), (2) CNS dysfunction (neurological impairment; cognitive or developmental delay), and (3) presence of at least two characteristic dysmorphic facial features.* Assist mother in providing adequate care and support her with praise for each accomplishment. *Nurturing of mother increases self-esteem and promotes nurturing of infant.* Facilitate access to well-child care. Assess home for safety hazards. Monitor compliance. *Because of the complex needs of both the FAS child and his/ her family, basic health and safety issues can be easily overlooked.*

*For the infant with fetal alcohol syndrome experiencing motor and mental impairment.

Growth and Development, Altered—cont'd

PATIENT GOALS/ EXPECTED OUTCOMES	NURSING INTERVENTIONS/ SCIENTIFIC RATIONALE
	Provide support and reinforce appropriate parenting activities; suggest ways to provide appropriate environment and stimulation based on infant's cues. *FAS infants have a higher incidence of irritability, abnormal sleep patterns, agitation, increased crying, and resistance to cuddling or holding. This behavior may frustrate parents, cause them to withdraw, or result in failure to thrive or abuse.*
	Monitor nutritional status: assess mother's feeding technique, provide guidance related to feeding problems, and assist/encourage mother to select foods that will provide calories and nutrition. *Although FAS infants have normal patterns of oral motor function, they have delays in the normal progression of oral feeding development. Many breastfeed poorly, have persistent vomiting and difficulty adjusting to solid foods, and show little interest in food.*

continued.

Growth and Development, Altered—cont'd

PATIENT GOALS/ EXPECTED OUTCOMES	NURSING INTERVENTIONS/ *SCIENTIFIC RATIONALE*
Achieve family adaptation as evidenced by the following: Obtains and uses appropriate supportive services	Make appropriate referrals to AA counselor for help with alcohol problem, social worker for financial or employment problems, early intervention program/physical therapist to support motor and cognitive development, nutritionist to ensure adequate caloric intake, and agency providing day care or respite care for special-needs children. Monitor family adaptation. Collaborate with involved professionals. *Care for FAS child is similar to care for children with other chronic conditions; needs are long-term; neurological problems continue through life-span and can include: delays in fine and gross motor, cognitive functioning, expressive and receptive language; vision deficits learning disabilities; psychosocial problems; difficulties in adaptive functioning.*

Growth and Development, Altered—cont'd

PATIENT GOALS/ EXPECTED OUTCOMES	NURSING INTERVENTIONS/ SCIENTIFIC RATIONALE
Increase mother's understanding of dangers of alcohol consumption during pregnancy as evidenced by the following: Prevent future FAS-affected births	Provide information about teratogenic effect of alcohol on fetus. *FAS is a leading cause of mental retardation and is preventable. "Safe" level of exposure of fetus to alcohol has not been determined. Therefore total abstinence during pregnancy is recommended.*

References 183, 307, 437, 610.

Health Maintenance, Altered

Related factors: Impaired ability to make deliberate and thoughtful judgments; insufficient material resources

Nancy Creason, Judy Minton, Kim Astroth, and Mi Ja Kim

PATIENT GOALS/ EXPECTED OUTCOMES	NURSING INTERVENTIONS/ *SCIENTIFIC RATIONALE*
Seek help as needed to maintain health as evidenced by the following:	
Clarifies health maintenance needs	Help patient to clarify health maintenance needs.
Defines type of help needed for health maintenance	Assist patient in defining what help is needed to maintain health.
	Assessment of patient's perceived risk factors can enhance relevant health maintenance behaviors.
Describes resources	Teach patient/significant others about helpful resources available in family, community, and so on. *Knowledge of resources facilitates action.*
Selects helping resources based on evaluation in relation to needs	Help patient to evaluate potential or actual effectiveness of available resources.
Contacts resources as appropriate	Support patient in establishing contact with appropriate resources.
Reports use of help as needed to maintain health	Help patient to clarify factors that impair ability to maintain health. *Active learning leads to more effective integration of knowledge.*
Consults with significant others in defining health maintenance needs	Support significant others with their role in helping patient maintain health. *Involving significant others can enhance and reinforce the practice of health maintenance behaviors.*

Health Maintenance, Altered—cont'd

PATIENT GOALS/ EXPECTED OUTCOMES	NURSING INTERVENTIONS/ *SCIENTIFIC RATIONALE*
Reestablish ability to maintain health as evidenced by the following:	
Identifies factors affecting present altered health maintenance ability	Help patient to evaluate personal strengths and weaknesses that affect health maintenance ability.
Recognizes personal strengths and weaknesses	
Uses strengths to reestablish health maintenance ability	Support patient in organizing and using strengths for health maintenance. *Individuals all have unique strengths that can be used to maintain health. Individual values will affect decision making.*
Works to improve problem-solving skills	Teach patient about the problem-solving process.
Uses community resources appropriately	Teach patient about community resources supportive of health maintenance practices.
	Monitor patient's progress in reestablishing health maintenance control. *Individuals can be helped to modify life-style and control health behaviors.*
Monitor and identify further health maintenance needs as evidenced by the following:	
Provides input about health maintenance activities	Monitor patient's ability to maintain health.
Reports awareness of altered health state	Educate patient to recognize altered health state.
Develops effective behavior to support health maintenance	Help patient to develop behaviors that support health maintenance. *A person's perspective of health, locus of control, self-esteem, and health status influence health prevention behavior.*

continued.

Health Maintenance, Altered—cont'd

PATIENT GOALS/ EXPECTED OUTCOMES	NURSING INTERVENTIONS/ *SCIENTIFIC RATIONALE*
Participates actively in health maintenance activities	Collaborate with patient to determine and develop behaviors needed to maintain health. *Interpersonal interactions support a person's tendency to be self-actualizing.*

References 65, 95, 105, 126, 127, 157, 179, 271, 451, 455.

Health-Seeking Behaviors (Stress Management)

Contextual factors: Desire for improved quality of life
Jane Lancour and Audrey M. McLane

PATIENT GOALS/ EXPECTED OUTCOMES	NURSING INTERVENTIONS/ SCIENTIFIC RATIONALE
Experience a trusting relationship as evidenced by the following:	
Identifies present state of wellness and areas in life-style that require attention	Introduce client to Travis Wellness Inventory and Crumbaugh and Maholick's Purpose in Life Test.
	Promote client's interest in completing Inventory and Life Test.
	Assist client in interpreting findings.
	Help client to identify factors that threaten personal wellness and action that can be taken.
	Discuss with client the interdependent and interactive relationship of present state of well-being to daily behaviors, thinking, attitudes, and beliefs.
Identifies realistic goals and plans for enhancing health	Facilitate verbalization of desire for change, fears, excitement, priorities, goals, and possible action.
Experience enhanced self-awareness as evidenced by the following:	
Verbalizes present patterns of response to stress and use of coping strategies	Assist client in identifying present stressors: internal processes and external events.
	Assist client in identifying behavioral responses to stress. *The immune system weakens under conditions of chronic stress, increasing susceptibility to illness.*

continued.

Health-Seeking Behaviors (Stress Management)—cont'd

PATIENT GOALS/ EXPECTED OUTCOMES	NURSING INTERVENTIONS/ *SCIENTIFIC RATIONALE*
	Explore client's use of coping strategies and degree of effectiveness.
	Assist client in assessing quality of dietary intake and physical activity program. Share with client the relationship of nutritional status, exercise, and stress management.
	Examine with client the feasibility of using conscious relaxation as a means of taking positive personal control. *Learning internally-oriented relaxation techniques (e.g., autogenic training or meditation) helps patient gain/maintain a sense of control.*
Consistently engages in one self-training approach. Communicates outcomes of engaging in program(s) of choice and modifies approach as desired	Elicit client's willingness and interest in expanding self-awareness through self-training programs: self-hypnosis, creative visualization, meditation, sound therapy, and so on.
	Share with client the process of integrating selected/desired programs. Provide client with follow-up resource material.
	Emphasize importance of consistency, patience, working within unique capacity in carrying out self-training program.

References 133, 516, 589.

Home Maintenance Management, Impaired

Related factors: Inadequate knowledge about postoperative home management; impaired mobility status*

Marie Maguire, Linda K. Young, Marilyn Harter, and Audrey M. McLane

PATIENT GOALS/ EXPECTED OUTCOMES	NURSING INTERVENTIONS/ SCIENTIFIC RATIONALE
Integrate hip precautions into ADLs as evidenced by the following:	
Avoids extreme flexion of hip more than 90 degrees (e.g., avoids bending from hip; uses elevated toilet seat)	Collaborate with physical therapist about hip precaution teaching. *An interdisciplinary approach enhances teaching.*
Avoids adduction of hip (e.g., avoids crossing legs)	Use written instructions to reinforce learning about hip precautions. *Written instructions ensure a consistent resource.*
Avoids internal rotation of hip (e.g., uses abduction wedge or pillows between legs when lying in bed)	Monitor integration of hip precautions into performance of ADLs as independence progressively increases *to ensure that patient incorporates teaching into practice.*
	Monitor progress and compliance with treatment plan. *Monitoring provides evaluation and gives direction for additional teaching.*
	Instruct patient about signs and symptoms of dislocation *to ensure that patient has knowledge of potential complications.*
Progress toward independence in ADLs as evidenced by the following:	
Manages personal hygiene with assistance of home health aide three times per week	
Correctly and consistently uses assistive devices to facilitate ADLs	Encourage use of assistive devices *to promote safe healing of hip.*

*For patient with total hip replacement, posterior approach.

continued.

HOME MAINTENANCE MANAGEMENT, IMPAIRED

PATIENT GOALS/ EXPECTED OUTCOMES	NURSING INTERVENTIONS/ *SCIENTIFIC RATIONALE*
Alternates periods of activity and rest	
Eats a balanced diet	
Participates actively in performance of ADLs with less assistance over time	Foster gradual independence in ADLs. *Attaining maximal independence fosters successful reintegration into home environment.*
	Teach patient to pace activities *to enhance healing of involved hip joint and muscle.*
Verbalizes knowledge of treatment plan and community resources.	Teach patient proper use of pain medication and side effects.
Selects/participates in one outside activity per week.	Encourage progressive increase in activities inside/outside the home (with physician approval). *Progressive activity increase allows for healing and strengthening.*
	Collaborate with patient/significant other to arrange for home health services (e.g., home health aide and/or registered nurse). *Such services promote return to independent living situation.*
	Collaborate with patient/significant other or household member to arrange for continuing rehabilitative services (e.g., physical therapy provided in outpatient department or in the home setting). *These services promote return to independent living situation.*
	Arrange for Meals on Wheels *to provide nutritional support necessary for optimal healing.*

Home Maintenance Management, Impaired—cont'd

PATIENT GOALS/ EXPECTED OUTCOMES	NURSING INTERVENTIONS/ *SCIENTIFIC RATIONALE*
Plan for adapting home environment to promote maximal health and safety as evidenced by the following:	
Verbalizes plan for moving excess furniture to clear pathway for walker.	Collaborate with patient/significant other to plan for a safe home environment. *Mutual planning enhances compliance.*
Identifies need to remove loose scatter rugs.	Assist patient in negotiating rental/purchase and installation of bathtub rails, tub bench, elevated toilet seat, and grab bars. *Using such items promotes independence and safety with ADLs.*
Consistently and correctly uses safety aids in bathroom (e.g., tub rails, elevated toilet seat, grab bars, tub bench)	
	Encourage patient to wear nonskid shoes *to enhance safe mobility.*
	Instruct patient to use chair with firm seat and armrests. *Such furniture maintains correct hip alignment at no more than 90 degrees flexion and facilitates safe transfer activities.*
Uses utility bag attached to walker for miscellaneous supplies (e.g., cordless telephone)	Encourage use of cordless telephone *to ensure ability to summon emergency assistance.*
Identifies need to maintain a well-lighted environment (e.g., keeps hall and bathroom lights on at night)	Instruct patient to keep environment well lighted *to enhance safe mobility.*
Significant other/household members express satisfaction with home maintenance	Provide patient/significant other or household member with 24-hour emergency number for health services *to ensure ability to summon emergency assistance.*

References 11, 258, 428, 445, 476, 485, 579, 630.

Hopelessness

Related factors: Isolation from prolonged activity restriction*
Charlotte E. Naschinski and Gertrude K. McFarland

PATIENT GOALS/ EXPECTED OUTCOMES	NURSING INTERVENTIONS/ *SCIENTIFIC RATIONALE*
Reduce isolation from environment as evidenced by the following:	
Maintains relationships with others	Establish contact and rapport with patient.
Participates in diversional activities	Assist patient in identifying enjoyable diversional activities.
Establishes a support network	Provide opportunities for patient to spend time with one other person; gradually increase amount of time and number of persons.
	Discuss with patient options for increasing support networks.
Reports satisfaction from relationships with others	Encourage visits by others.
	Hope depends on interaction with significant others and thrives in an atmosphere of trust.
Express feelings as evidenced by the following:	
Identifies feelings	Provide opportunity for patient to express feelings verbally or nonverbally (e.g., writing or drawing).
Expresses feelings both verbally and nonverbally	Facilitate expression of feelings by active listening, open-ended questions, and reflection.
	Provide opportunity for physical expression of feelings (e.g., punching bag or exercises), when possible, and within physical capabilities.
	Express empathy while communicating belief that patient can act contrary to the way he/she feels.

*For the patient with chronic obstructive pulmonary disease and depression.

Hopelessness—cont'd

PATIENT GOALS/ EXPECTED OUTCOMES	NURSING INTERVENTIONS/ *SCIENTIFIC RATIONALE*
	Offer realistic hope through communicating belief that patient has or can learn skills needed to cope with problems and physical limitations.
	Assist patient in identifying person(s) with whom he/she is comfortable sharing feelings.
Reports absence of suicidal ideation	Observe for signs of suicidal intent (e.g., sudden behavior or mood change, conversations about futility of life).
	Expressing feelings abates hopelessness.
Increase self-confidence as evidenced by the following:	
Reports increased feelings of self-worth	Demonstrate unconditional positive regard for patient.
Identifies strengths and abilities	Assist patient in identifying those roles that can consistently be carried out successfully within physical limitations.
Maintains good grooming and personal hygiene habits	Assist patient in developing self-care skills that contribute to mastery of environment.
	Encourage patient to identify and participate in satisfying experiences.
	Encourage positive self-statements by patient.
	Provide honest praise about patient's accomplishments.
	Developing self-confidence depends on repetitive positive interactions and mastery of the environment.

continued.

Hopelessness—cont'd

PATIENT GOALS/ EXPECTED OUTCOMES	NURSING INTERVENTIONS/ *SCIENTIFIC RATIONALE*
Control or influence self and environment as evidenced by the following:	
Verbalizes ability to control or influence self and environment	Encourage independent behavior. Involve patient in decisions about ADLs and health care. Teach patient how to discriminate between controllable and uncontrollable events.
Identifies realistic goals	Assist patient in determining realistic goals.
Demonstrates effective coping strategies	Assist patient in identifying alternative ways to cope. Assist patient in identifying consequences of implementing identified alternatives. Teach patient new coping strategies.
Uses effective communication techniques	Demonstrate and teach effective communication techniques (e.g., active listening).
Demonstrates effective problem-solving skills Reports finding meaning in life	*The perception of control over self and the environment is enhanced through expanding the patient's ability to cope, problem-solve, and communicate.*

References 78, 171, 355, 417, 563, 606.

Hyperthermia

Related factor: Exposure to hot environment*
Kathryn Czurylo and Mi Ja Kim

PATIENT GOALS/ EXPECTED OUTCOMES	NURSING INTERVENTIONS/ *SCIENTIFIC RATIONALE*
Maintain normothermia as evidenced by the following: Absence of hyperthermia signs and symptoms, such as tachycardia, hyperventilation, flushed skin, and seizures Normothermia Respiration, pulse, and blood pressure within normal limits for patient	Monitor temperature and vital signs every hour. Apply internal/external cooling measures as appropriate, such as cool sponge bath or cooling mattress. *When using cooling mattress, bring temperature down gradually to prevent shivering as much as possible because it causes increased oxygen consumption.* Provide IV fluid therapy per order. Provide fluids, 3000 ml/24 hours or as ordered. *Dehydration may be present due to loss of fluid from diaphoresis and increased ventilation.* Monitor arterial blood gas levels and blood and urine lab tests and report abnormalities. Administer antipyretics as ordered. Provide temperature-controlled, comfortable environment.

*For the patient with heat stroke.
References 76, 260, 338, 341.

202

Hypothermia

Related factor: Exposure to cold environment*
Kathryn Czurylo and Mi Ja Kim

PATIENT GOALS/ EXPECTED OUTCOMES	NURSING INTERVENTIONS/ SCIENTIFIC RATIONALE
Maintain normothermia as evidenced by the following:	
Absence of signs and symptoms of hypothermia: shivering, cool skin, pallor	Slowly rewarm body by internal/external methods as appropriate (e.g., administer room temperature or warmed IV solution per order/may wrap extremities using towels to control shivering).
Normothermia	
Pulse, respiration, and blood pressure within normal limits for patient	
Warm skin	Monitor temperature using low-reading thermometer.
	Monitor vital signs every hour; monitor ECG continuously; report arrhythmias, such as bradycardia, and treat per order. *During hypothermia, circulating volume decreases, causing decreased cardiac output and resulting in decreased oxygen delivery and arrhythmias.*
	Monitor arterial blood gases levels. *Because of medullary respiratory depression, respiratory acidosis may result.*
	Monitor lab values; serum electrolytes, BUN, creatinine, glucose, and CBC and report abnormalities. *Endocrine, liver, and renal functions decrease as temperature decreases; WBC and platelet count may decrease as a result of sequestration in spleen, liver, and vascular beds.*

*For the patient with cold injury.

Hypothermia—cont'd

PATIENT GOALS/ EXPECTED OUTCOMES	NURSING INTERVENTIONS/ *SCIENTIFIC RATIONALE*
	Insert indwelling catheter per order and monitor urine output every 30 minutes *to assess body fluid balance and renal function.* Provide temperature-controlled, comfortable environment.

References 30, 101, 145, 165, 238, 253, 264, 341, 439, 640.

INCONTINENCE, FUNCTIONAL

Related factors: Restricted mobility requiring use of equipment or device; on prescribed diuretic; no established toileting regimen

Audrey M. McLane and Ruth E. McShane

PATIENT GOALS/ EXPECTED OUTCOMES	NURSING INTERVENTIONS/ *SCIENTIFIC RATIONALE*
Achieve continence as evidenced by the following:	
Gradual decrease in episodes of incontinence	Teach progressive use of Kegel's exercises.[543 p. 215]
Keeps a log to record episodes of involuntary loss of urine	
Responds to positive reinforcement	Provide positive feedback in conjunction with incontinence checks.
Establish/adhere to toileting routine as evidenced by the following:	
Attempts voiding every 1 hour and gradually increases to every 3 to 4 hours.	Establish 1-hour prompted voiding schedule; gradually increase to 3 to 4 hours if tolerated.
Voids before retiring	
Uses voiding log to record changes in pattern of urination	Teach/monitor use of voiding record to document voiding attempts.
Modify environment to facilitate continence as evidenced by the following:	
Accepts use of commode	Provide patient with list of resources to rent/purchase commode.
Designates private area for use of commode	Assist patient with selection and creation of private area for commode and supplies on first floor of residence. *Private area for use of commode will facilitate patient-initiated voiding attempts.*
Keeps walking aids and supplies nearby	
Uses continence aids to protect skin and clothing	
Wears clothing easy to manage for toileting	
Keeps lights on in upstairs hallway and bathroom at night	Encourage placement of extra telephone near commode.

Incontinence, Functional—cont'd

PATIENT GOALS/ EXPECTED OUTCOMES	NURSING INTERVENTIONS/ *SCIENTIFIC RATIONALE*
Establish/adhere to diuretic and fluid intake routine as evidenced by the following: Takes afternoon diuretic 4 to 5 hours before bedtime Drinks 8 oz of liquid with meals, between meals, and 2 to 3 hours before bedtime	Develop with patient a schedule for taking diuretics and fluids. Monitor medications for drugs that influence bladder tone and/or amount of urine production. Determine consistency of use of K^+ supplement of foods high in K^+. *Low K^+ level decreases bladder tone.*
Reestablish social contacts with friends and family as evidenced by the following: Leaves home for 1- to 2-hour periods to visit family/friends Gradually returns to usual social activities	Plan with patient and family for short trips away from residence. Demonstrate sensitivity to patient's feelings about incontinence episodes. Encourage use of continence aids to protect clothing. *Use of continence aids when away from home will alleviate patient's anxiety and contribute to continence.*

References 363, 433, 543, 592, 600.

INCONTINENCE, REFLEX

Related factor: Spinal cord lesion above the level of the reflex arc*

Audrey M. McLane and Ruth E. McShane

PATIENT GOALS/ EXPECTED OUTCOMES	NURSING INTERVENTIONS/ *SCIENTIFIC RATIONALE*
Achieve continence as evidenced by the following:	
Expresses willingness to try manual voiding techniques	Assist in selection, teaching, and trial of manual voiding facilitation techniques (e.g., stimulation of anus, tapping lower abdomen, doing push-ups on commode). *A reflex bladder contraction occurs in response to perineal or lower abdominal stimulation.*
Participates in selection of cues/reminders to void	Establish cues/reminders to void.
	Monitor amount of residual urine.
Patient/significant other participate in learning clean intermittent catheterization (CIC)	Demonstrate and have patient/significant other return demonstrate CIC. *Patient/significant other must learn CIC to monitor residual urine; knowing CIC gives patient greater sense of control.*
Episodes of incontinence rare	
	Determine need for use of urinary containment device at night.
	Establish a catheterization schedule, usually every 4 to 6 hours.
	Determine patient's understanding of role of medications (autonomic or spasmolytic) in maintaining continence.
Maintain renal function as evidenced by the following:	
Urinalysis confirms absence of infection	Teach/monitor use of appropriate hygienic measures (e.g., washing hands and perineum before procedure).

*For the patient with absence of nerve pathways to brain but intact sacral spinal reflexes.

Incontinence, Reflex—cont'd

PATIENT GOALS/ EXPECTED OUTCOMES	NURSING INTERVENTIONS/ *SCIENTIFIC RATIONALE*
	Teach patient/significant other how to clean/store catheters and other devices.
	Teach patient/significant other signs and symptoms of bladder/urinary tract infection.
	Monitor color, amount, and odor of urine.
	Establish written plan for fluid intake (e.g., 200 ml every 2 hrs).
	Teach use of fluid intake/output record.
Maintain skin integrity as evidenced by the following:	
Skin remains intact	Provide written plan to keep skin clean and dry.
	Monitor skin for signs of redness, abrasions, and so on.
Obtains/uses protective and easy-to-remove clothing	Provide information about protective and easy-to-remove clothing.

References 181, 216, 363, 533, 549, 600.

Incontinence, Stress

Related factors: Weak sphincter, pelvic muscles, and structural supports

Ruth E. McShane and Audrey M. McLane

PATIENT GOALS/ EXPECTED OUTCOMES	NURSING INTERVENTIONS/ *SCIENTIFIC RATIONALE*
Increase pelvic floor muscle tone and sphincter function as evidenced by the following:	
Performs pelvic floor exercises (PFEs) three times a day for 6 months	Teach patient a method for doing PFEs and provide written instructions: Sit or stand without tensing muscles of legs, buttocks, or abdomen. Contract and relax circumvaginal muscles and urinary and anal sphincters for 3 to 4 seconds and repeat in a staccato fashion. Do PFE 25 to 30 times, three times a daily. *PFEs strengthen the circumvaginal muscles, urinary sphincter, and external anal sphincter.*
Reduce incontinence episodes as evidenced by the following:	
Keeps voiding record	Teach patient to keep voiding log. Monitor number and pattern of incontinence episodes.
Uses timer to provide cue to void every 2 hours	Instruct patient to void by the clock, beginning with 2-hour intervals. Instruct patient to lengthen interval between voidings gradually.
Drinks 6 to 8 glasses of water a day	Assist patient in establishing fluid intake pattern to maintain hydration (e.g., 200 ml every 2 hours during day).

Incontinence, Stress—cont'd

PATIENT GOALS/ EXPECTED OUTCOMES	NURSING INTERVENTIONS/ *SCIENTIFIC RATIONALE*
Increase in self-esteem and social functioning as evidenced by the following:	
	Provide positive reinforcement for desired behaviors. Teach use of continence aids. Assist with development of plan for participation in outside activities.
Participates in social/recreational activities on a regular basis	

References 159, 215a, 349, 363, 549, 600.

INCONTINENCE, TOTAL

Related factor: Anatomic (fistula)*
Ruth E. McShane and Audrey M. McLane

PATIENT GOALS/ EXPECTED OUTCOMES	NURSING INTERVENTIONS/ *SCIENTIFIC RATIONALE*
Achieve a schedule of complete, regular bladder evacuation as evidenced by the following:	
Incontinent episodes are contained	Provide urinary containment device for immediate use *because most routine treatment modalities are ineffective.*
	Determine origin of urine loss (urethra, vagina, other).
	Identify conditions that increase or decrease urine loss.
Avoid urological complications as evidenced by the following:	
Makes and keeps appointment with urologist	Refer patient for medical evaluation.
	Monitor color, odor, and amount of urine.
Patient/caregiver returns demonstration of intermittent catheterization	Demonstrate/monitor clean intermittent catheterization *to prevent urinary infection.*
	Establish/implement written plan for fluid intake (e.g., 200 ml every 2 hours from 8 AM to 6 PM).
Maintain skin integrity as evidenced by the following:	
Skin remains intact	Develop/implement written plan for keeping skin clean/dry.
	Monitor skin for signs of redness, abrasions and so on.
	Demonstrate use of protective clothing.
	Provide information about easy-to-remove clothing.

*For the patient following trauma and surgery with self-care limitations, functional level 3.

Incontinence, Total—cont'd

PATIENT GOALS/ EXPECTED OUTCOMES	NURSING INTERVENTIONS/ *SCIENTIFIC RATIONALE*
Achieve desired level of independence in self-care as evidenced by the following:	
Monitors own fluid intake/voiding patterns and makes adjustments	Teach use of voiding record.
Sets goals for increase in self-care ability	Establish plan to gain independence in self-care consistent with limitations.
Patient/caregiver identifies problems/potential problems related to use of urinary containment devices.	Develop with patient/caregiver strategies for coping with use of urinary containment devices.
Maintain patient's/caregiver's dignity and feelings of self-worth as evidenced by the following:	
Increase in number of positive self-statements	Monitor nurse/patient interactions for negative statements about self.
	Teach patient thought-stopping and thought-substitution techniques.
	Use behavioral approaches acceptable to patient and caregiver.
Primary caregiver participates in outside recreational/social activities weekly	Evaluate caregiver's perceived health, sense of well-being, and feelings/of burden.
	Discuss with patient/caregiver importance of planning for caregiver's participation in desired recreational/social activities.

References 110, 198, 216, 363, 507, 533, 600.

Related factors: History of recurrent bladder infections; high caffeine intake

Audrey M. McLane and Ruth E. McShane

PATIENT GOALS/ EXPECTED OUTCOMES	NURSING INTERVENTIONS/ *SCIENTIFIC RATIONALE*
Modify diet and fluid intake to maintain adequate acid of urine as evidenced by the following:	
Drinks concentrated cranberry juice daily	Teach patient to drink concentrated cranberry juice and/or take superphysiological doses of vitamin C. *In very large doses, vitamin C is not metabolized and is excreted in urine as ascorbic acid. The acidity of urine helps to prevent bacterial growth.*
Takes superphysiological amounts of vitamin C	
Drinks 8 oz of fluid with each meal, between meals, and in early evening	Teach patient to drink 8 oz of liquid with meals, between meals, and in early evening.
Substitutes herbal teas for regular teas.	Teach patient to decrease ingestion of caffeine-containing liquids.
Establish/adhere to toileting routine as evidenced by the following:	
Attempts voiding every 2 hours, with gradual increase to every 3 to 4 hours	Assist patient with development of toileting routine.
	Teach/monitor use of voiding record.
Uses pelvic floor exercises regularly to strengthen muscles	Teach pelvic floor exercises.
Uses voiding log to record voiding attempts, practice of pelvic floor exercises, and episodes of incontinence	Monitor/evaluate change in voiding pattern.
Voids before retiring	

Incontinence, Urge—cont'd

PATIENT GOALS/ EXPECTED OUTCOMES	NURSING INTERVENTIONS/ *SCIENTIFIC RATIONALE*
Alter pattern of response to urge to void as evidenced by the following:	
Avoids rushing to toilet	Teach patient to alter pattern of response to urge to void, including avoiding rushing to toilet; responding to urge to void by pausing to relax abdominal muscles; and proceeding at normal pace. *Relaxation of abdominal muscles decreases sense of urgency and helps patient remain continent.*
Responds to urge to void by pausing and relaxing abdominal muscles, then proceeding at a normal pace	
Reestablish continence as evidenced by the following:	
Episodes of involuntary loss of urine decrease	Provide positive feedback for small decreases in episodes of incontinence.
Uses measures to prevent recurrence of bladder infections (e.g., adequate fluid intake, superphysiological doses of vitamin C)	Teach patient to continue use of superphysiological doses of vitamin C and fluid intake schedule to prevent recurrence of urinary tract infection.
Absence of urinary tract infection as confirmed by urinalysis	Instruct patient to take antibiotics as prescribed.
	Teach patient to obtain midstream urine specimen at first sign of return of symptoms.

References 31, 88, 292, 363, 543, 549, 600.

Related factor: Prematurity
Emma B. Nemivant and Mi Ja Kim

PATIENT GOALS/ EXPECTED OUTCOMES	NURSING INTERVENTIONS/ *SCIENTIFIC RATIONALE*
For mother, recognize the methods to deliver expressed mother's milk (EMM) to the high-risk preterm infant as evidenced by the following: Knows why gavage method is to be used Knows the types of gavage feeding **For infant, achieve adequate nutritional state as evidenced by the following:** Gains weight Grows within expected limits	Provide information to the mother that most small, preterm infants cannot be breastfed directly. Therefore they receive EMM by artificial feeding such as gavage infusion until they have demonstrated the ability to feed orally. *Preterm infant's ability to coordinate sucking, swallowing, and breathing varies from 32 to 36 weeks of gestation, depending on feeding method.* Discuss possible adverse, short-term, physiological, and biochemical responses to intermittent bolus gavage feeding; such as apnea, bradycardia, and hypoxemia *to determine whether to use continuous or intermittent gavage feeding.*

Infant Feeding Pattern, Ineffective—cont'd

PATIENT GOALS/ EXPECTED OUTCOMES	NURSING INTERVENTIONS/ *SCIENTIFIC RATIONALE*
	Use intermittent bolus gavage infusion of EMM at a slow rate for all preterm infants whenever possible *to minimize or prevent adverse sequelae of rapid gastric filling.*
	Administer EMM by continuous nasogastric (CNG) infusion, if needed, by using following safeguards:
	Perform routine bacteriologic surveillance of EMM *so that EMM contains only skin flora in concentration not exceeding 10^3 colony-forming units (cfu) per ml.*
	Infuse the EMM at the highest possible rate that is safe for the infant *to minimize the bacterial growth and nutrient loss.*
	Use syringe pump placed at 45-degree angle and small-lumen infusion tubing *to minimize nutrient loss.*
	Measure lipid content of EMM by creamatocrit at the distal end of the infusion system. *If lipid adheres to the infusion syringe and tubing, infants may receive a more dilute, low-calorie milk and subsequently demonstrate suboptimal growth.*
	Change syringe and tubing every 4 hours *to minimize bacterial growth.*

References 70, 109, 240, 365, 381, 382, 384, 385, 386.

Risk factor: Suppressed immune system*
Kathryn Czurylo and Mi Ja Kim

PATIENT GOALS/ EXPECTED OUTCOMES	NURSING INTERVENTIONS/ *SCIENTIFIC RATIONALE*
Experience no infection as evidenced by the following: Negative culture WBC within normal limits for patient Afebrile Other vital signs within normal limits for patient Patient/significant other verbalizes knowledge of infection prevention	Monitor temperature every 4 hours; report elevation. Auscultate lungs daily; have patient report sore throat or perianal tenderness. *Typical signs of inflammation may be absent in neutropenia.* Weigh patient daily. Check body fluids for alterations in color, odor, or consistency. Teach patient to choose high-calorie, high-protein, high-vitamin foods. *Such foods will promote cellular repair and regeneration and help produce lymphocytes.* Follow steps for prevention of impaired skin integrity. Limit use of aspirin/acetaminophen *because these may mask a fever.* Encourage daily shower/good oral hygiene. Encourage fluids, 2600 ml/day. Obtain cultures per order and report abnormalities. Monitor results of CBC and report WBC abnormalities. *Neutropenia of 500-1000 increases risk of infection.* Wash hands before each contact with patient. Use gloves as necessary. Discontinue invasive lines as soon as possible. Avoid invasive procedures.

*For the patient with cancer chemotherapy–induced immunosuppression.

Infection, High Risk for—cont'd

PATIENT GOALS/ EXPECTED OUTCOMES	NURSING INTERVENTIONS/ *SCIENTIFIC RATIONALE*
	Use strict aseptic technique when performing invasive procedures. Prevent patient exposure to infected visitors/staff. Use reverse isolation if indicated. Teach patient/significant other above interventions when appropriate.

References 96, 114, 218, 223, 229, 257, 490, 495.

INJURY, HIGH RISK FOR

Risk factors: Emotional lability; cognitive impairment*
Gertrude K. McFarland and Karen E. Inaba

PATIENT GOALS/ EXPECTED OUTCOMES	NURSING INTERVENTIONS/ SCIENTIFIC RATIONALE
Not injure self as evidenced by the following:	
Demonstrates impulse control and appropriate judgment, and remains free from personal injury	Foster interpersonal trust.
	Identify personal or environmental risk factors *to assess and quantify safety needs and level of vulnerability.*
	Monitor emotional state (e.g., depression, anxiety, anger, suspiciousness) *to determine level of arousal and early signs of escalation.*
	Evaluate degree of cognitive impairment.
	Monitor judgment, decision-making ability, and impulse control *to determine amount of surveillance needed.*
	Examine physical environment for possible risks and remove hazardous objects or make modifications in setting, as necessary, *to promote safety.*
Recognizes stressors that may increase risk of injury	Assist in identifying stressors within patient or the environment *to obtain patient's perception of threat and to assess coping capacity.*
Seeks protective environment when needed.	Monitor stress levels (observation and patient self-report).
	Reduce environmental overstimulation (e.g., excessive noise), crowding, invasion of personal space, frustrating situations, and so on, *to minimize sense of threat.*
	Avoid power struggles between staff and patient by permitting reasonable choices.

*For the patient with borderline personality disorder.

Injury, High Risk for—cont'd

PATIENT GOALS/ EXPECTED OUTCOMES	NURSING INTERVENTIONS/ *SCIENTIFIC RATIONALE*
	Determine appropriate interpersonal distance and nonverbal communication *to prevent anxiety and defensive responses.*
	Determine limits and maintain consistency.
	Administer medications to calm patient, if appropriate.
	Evaluate social network and role of significant others in affecting patient's behavior. *Social pressure and support may facilitate positive coping and reinforce appropriate responses.*
	Plan for unpredictable dangerous behaviors toward self or others.
Identifies moods that may increase risk of injury	Encourage expression of feelings *to decrease tension and anxiety.*
Engages in constructive activities that channel emotions	Teach patient about self-monitoring emotional state in self *to promote greater awareness of personal threshold for stress.*
Maintains control of own behavior	
Uses previous constructive and recently learned strategies to cope with stress	Teach patient constructive physical and mental strategies to channel emotions *to provide outlets for tension and appropriate release of energy.*
Seeks appropriate therapies and community resources as needed	Teach patient stress-management techniques.
	As appropriate, refer to individual or group psychotherapy, support group, counseling, or other resources.
	Assist patient in planning and rehearsing coping strategies *to maintain control.*

continued.

PATIENT GOALS/ EXPECTED OUTCOMES	NURSING INTERVENTIONS/ *SCIENTIFIC RATIONALE*
	Assess suicidal risk *to determine need for increased surveillance.*
	Contract with patient about desired responses to stressors and acceptable behaviors (e.g., "no-harm" contract) *to facilitate consistency and clarification of therapeutic goals.*

References 50, 168, 233, 311, 346, 406, 461, 516, 516a, 524a.

Knowledge Deficit (Home IV Therapy)

Related factors: New experience; delayed readiness for learning

Jane Lancour and Audrey M. McLane

PATIENT GOALS/ EXPECTED OUTCOMES	NURSING INTERVENTIONS/ *SCIENTIFIC RATIONALE*
Develop trusting/helping relationship as evidenced by the following:	
Discusses with caregiver fears and concerns about health state, previous experiences with health care delivery, and therapeutic regimen	Allow sufficient time during each visit for one-to-one interaction. Sit quietly with patient and engage in active listening. Inform patient about time of each scheduled daily visit.
Calls caregiver with questions Seeks assistance/direction for financial insecurities	Instruct patient as to caregiver's availability via phone, between visits, and types of concerns/questions that could be discussed. Leave contact person's name for patient to call about financial information. Document patient's phone calls: time, date, content, and action taken. Capitalize on opportunities to compliment and/or praise.
Develop readiness for learning as evidenced by the following:	
Identifies past pattern of effective learning	Determine competency and comprehension potential for home IV therapy.
Seeks information through active dialogue	Monitor readiness to learn at each visit and determine best methods for teaching/learning. *Certain aspects of current/ongoing health situation may alter a patient's ability to learn/ retain information.*

continued.

Knowledge Deficit (Home IV Therapy)—cont'd

KNOWLEDGE DEFICIT (HOME IV THERAPY)

PATIENT GOALS/ EXPECTED OUTCOMES	NURSING INTERVENTIONS/ *SCIENTIFIC RATIONALE*
Uses printed information pieces as reinforcement to learning	Provide specific printed instructions (including pictures) for home IV therapy. Establish best approach for teaching: structured, unstructured, or both. Use patient teaching flow sheet.
Increase knowledge and skill of basic IV therapy as evidenced by the following:	
	Evaluate home setting for an area to store supplies and for preparing solutions.
Demonstrates handwashing procedure and use of aseptic technique	Demonstrate and have patient return demonstration on handwashing technique and aseptic technique. Inspect site of IV puncture at each visit.
Demonstrates correct preparation of IV fluids (i.e., bag labeling, attaching tubing, and clearing the line)	Label needle device with data, time, size, and length of catheter. Change tubing every 48 hours. Complete site care every 48 hours. Demonstrate and have patient return demonstration on how to add IV solution. Demonstrate and have patient return demonstration on use of infusion pump.
Demonstrates correct discontinuance of IV fluid Demonstrates correct method of capping line	Demonstrate and have patient return demonstration on discontinuance of IV solution and capping of line.
Disposes of equipment as demonstrated	Evaluate patient's disposal of IV equipment. Demonstrate disposal of IV equipment in home setting.
Demonstrates correct recording on IV sheet	Demonstrate method for recording IV therapy.

Knowledge Deficit (Home IV Therapy)—cont'd

PATIENT GOALS/ EXPECTED OUTCOMES	NURSING INTERVENTIONS/ *SCIENTIFIC RATIONALE*
	Evaluate entries made by patient on IV record. *Teaching/learning effectiveness is enhanced when patient becomes actively engaged in the learning process.*
Offset potential complications as evidenced by the following:	
Identifies signs and symptoms of infiltration and phlebitis	Describe signs and symptoms of infiltration and how it occurs. Describe signs and symptoms of phlebitis and basis of its occurrence.
Verbalizes action to take if evidence of infiltration or phlebitis is noted	Instruct in action to be taken if evidence of either infiltration or phlebitis is noted.
Checks IV site and flow rate every 2 hours during infusion	Instruct patient to check IV site and flow rate every 2 hours.
Verbalizes rationale for regulation of flow	
Verbalizes action to take if uncertain about events	

References 80a, 108, 192, 192a, 479, 485, 488.

Management of Therapeutic Regimen (Individuals), Ineffective

Related factors: Perceived barriers; perceived benefits; powerlessness

Joan M. Caley and Gertrude K. McFarland

PATIENT GOALS/ EXPECTED OUTCOMES	NURSING INTERVENTIONS/ *SCIENTIFIC RATIONALE*
Make effective choices in ADLs and achieve goals of treatment program as evidenced by the following:	
Decreased feelings of powerlessness	Evaluate patient's attitudes, values, and beliefs about current health state and treatment regimen.
Increases sense of control in making choices about treatment program	Evaluate impact of disease state/treatment regimen on current life-style and level of function.
Overcomes perceived barriers	Explore with patient past experiences, strengths, problems in illness, threats to health, and other stressful situations in which patient experiences feelings of powerlessness.
Recognizes and accepts benefits of treatment	
Meets goals of treatment program	Identify barriers that prevent the patient from engaging in treatment plan and feeling a sense of control over outcomes.
	Discuss with patient his/her perspectives on his/her future health status and life-style.
	It is important to determine patient's perspectives of current health status and treatment regimen to collaborate with patient in developing a practical plan for participating in treatment and meeting treatment goals.
	Teach patient about disease, illness manifestation, treatment plan, and goals for improved health status.

Management of Therapeutic Regimen (Individuals), Ineffective—cont'd

PATIENT GOALS/ EXPECTED OUTCOMES	NURSING INTERVENTIONS/ SCIENTIFIC RATIONALE
	Discuss with patient consequences of not adhering to treatment regimen and possible negative outcomes. *Adequate understanding of illness, involvement in treatment regimen, and outcomes serves as a baseline for developing a plan for behavioral change.*
	Provide feedback to patient on assessment of/and options that he/she might choose *to increase feelings of control and adherence to treatment regimen.*
	Collaborate with patient to develop plan in focusing on selected areas *to maximize patient's feelings of control. Capitalizing on strengths and starting with selected behavioral target areas for change are important beginning steps in developing a plan to participate effectively in treatment plan and meeting specific health goals.*
	Encourage patient to focus on single area and set small goals for a "trial period" to obtain feedback on how to be successful in his/her plan.
	Support patient in setting short-term manageable and achievable goals *to reach ultimate, long-range goals.*

continued.

Management of Therapeutic Regimen (Individuals), Ineffective—cont'd

PATIENT GOALS/ EXPECTED OUTCOMES	NURSING INTERVENTIONS/ *SCIENTIFIC RATIONALE*
	Support patient as he/she begins with plan, giving positive feedback and focusing on small achievements. *Small achievements and reaching short-term goals will decrease patient's sense of powerlessness and increase a sense of control over his/her health status and involvement in the treatment plan.* Refer patient to support groups that have a similar focus as patient and will provide positive reinforcement. *Careful selection of support groups is essential to avoid placing patient in situation with unrealistic expectations and that could have adverse outcomes on his/her feelings of content and achievement.* Encourage patient to discuss and seek out additional resources that will help him/her get positive feedback on adherence to treatment regimen and enhance his/her feelings of content and achievement.

Management of Therapeutic Regimen (Individuals), Ineffective—cont'd

PATIENT GOALS/ EXPECTED OUTCOMES	NURSING INTERVENTIONS/ *SCIENTIFIC RATIONALE*
	Monitor patient's progress at regular, scheduled intervals. Encourage patient to discuss progress, even setbacks. Reinforce setting manageable, achievable short-term goals for next interval. *Management of chronic illness requires the nurse to keep in mind long-range planning and goals, while focusing care planning with patient on more short-term, achievable goals that will contribute to the patient's ultimate long-term success.*

References 83, 309, 339, 398, 483, 564.

MOBILITY, IMPAIRED PHYSICAL

Related factors: Acute and chronic joint pain; fatigue*
Teresa Fadden, Janet F. Schulte, and Audrey M. McLane

PATIENT GOALS/ EXPECTED OUTCOMES	NURSING INTERVENTIONS/ SCIENTIFIC RATIONALE
Improve pain management as evidenced by the following:	
Rates pain as 3 or less on a scale of 10 over a 48-hour period	Teach patient how to use progressive relaxation as an adjunct to analgetics prn and at bedtime. *Pain control is a major component in maintaining optimal muscle and joint mobility.* Apply warm moist heat to affected joints. Provide warm showers prn and at bedtime to promote comfort. Avoid excessively hot water, *because this may increase fatigue.*
Self-administers prescribed antiinflammatory and/or analgetic medications consistently and on schedule	Teach appropriate use of antiinflammatory medications and analgetics, *which are most effective when administered on a consistent and fixed schedule to maintain adequate serum levels.*
Reports a minimum of 7 hours of uninterupted sleep for 3 consecutive days	Provide egg-crate mattress or similar joint-cushioning material for patient's bed to increase comfort. Suggest back massage at bedtime to promote sleep. Counsel patient to limit naps to no more than two a day. *Excessive napping during the day can interfere with normal sleep patterns.*

*For the patient with systemic lupus erythematosus.

Mobility, Impaired Physical—cont'd

PATIENT GOALS/ EXPECTED OUTCOMES	NURSING INTERVENTIONS/ *SCIENTIFIC RATIONALE*
	Monitor patient's emotional response to disease process, *because emotional state may have an impact on patient's ability to manage pain.*
Protect currently affected (acute) joints while promoting/maintaining function of joints affected by chronic lupus symptoms as evidenced by the following:	
Maintains full ROM in chronically affected joints	Coach patient through passive ROM before initiating active ROM twice daily to all but acutely affected joints to ensure safety and efficiency.
Rests and supports acutely affected joints	Provide rest and support to acutely affected joints *to stabilize and reduce stress on the joint and aid in muscle relaxation.*
	Splint inflamed wrists and hands. *Splinting can decrease pain by immobilizing the joint, and prevent contractures from forming in nonfunctional positions.*
Maintains daily exercise regimen as prescribed by physician and/or physical therapist	Balance rest therapy with active physical exercise program *to promote strength and function and to minimize fatigue related to activity level.*
Achieve optimal level of physical mobility as evidenced by the following:	
Provides own daily self-care within limits of any existing physical disabilities	Assist patient with task analysis of daily activities.
	Teach patient how to use a walker and other assistive devices correctly.

continued.

MOBILITY, IMPAIRED PHYSICAL

PATIENT GOALS/ EXPECTED OUTCOMES	NURSING INTERVENTIONS/ *SCIENTIFIC RATIONALE*
Performs ADLs in manner that promotes joint conservation and protection	Provide information about task simplification, assistive devices, and other energy-conserving techniques. Identify resources within patient's social support systems, and in wider community, that may aid in meeting ADLs outside the bounds of patient's current physical abilities (e.g., assistance with housework and transportation).

References 129, 227, 256, 305, 364, 462, 642.

Noncompliance (Therapeutic Regimen)

Related factors: Complexity of exercise regimen; side effects of medication*

Audrey M. McLane

PATIENT GOALS/ EXPECTED OUTCOMES	NURSING INTERVENTIONS/ *SCIENTIFIC RATIONALE*
Integrate exercise prescription into ADLs as evidenced by the following:	
Records time/distance walked in exercise log	Collaborate with patient/significant other to develop/implement a weekly exercise (activity/rest) plan. Teach patient/significant other how to use exercise log.
Records joint pain on scale of 1-10 before/after exercise and adjusts time/distance walked up/down as appropriate Modifies activities that consistently increase pain	Teach patient/significant other use of visual analog scale to record joint pain. *Logging exercise and rest may increase compliance with activity/rest prescription.*
Establish/adhere to schedule for taking medications as evidenced by the following:	
Takes nonsteroidal antiinflammatory drugs (NSAIDs) with food	Collaborate with patient/significant other to develop/implement plan for taking medications. *Active participation in decision making about therapeutic regimen may increase compliance.*

*For the older adult with degenerative joint disease who is on exercise regimen.

continued.

PATIENT GOALS/ EXPECTED OUTCOMES	NURSING INTERVENTIONS/ *SCIENTIFIC RATIONALE*
Makes appointment with physician if/when dissatisfied with medication side-effects	Review side effects of medications (e.g., gastrointestinal irritation from NSAIDs).
Records medications taken/ missed and any side effects	Discourage patient from discontinuing medications without consulting physician.
	Teach patient/significant other to record medications taken/ missed.
Makes and keeps appointment to evaluate compliance with regimen	Make appointment to interview patient and conduct "pill count" to evaluate compliance with medication regimen. *Patient interview is the most accurate measure of compliance.*

References 119, 128, 470, 511, 512, 604, 618, 619.

Nutrition, Altered: Less Than Body Requirements

Related factors: Increased work of breathing; inadequate intake of nutrients in diet

Audrey M. McLane, Colleen O'Brien, and Sheila Olson

PATIENT GOALS/ EXPECTED OUTCOMES	NURSING INTERVENTIONS/ *SCIENTIFIC RATIONALE*
Stabilize weight and then gradually increase to at least 10% less than ideal weight as evidenced by the following:	
Weight stabilizes (acceptable immediate outcome)	Collaborate with patient to establish a scale of weight outcomes from most desirable to least desirable. *Active participation in nutritional well-being contributes to patient's perception of control of life.*
Achieve weight gain of 1 lb every 3 weeks, increasing to 1 lb every 2 weeks (most desirable outcome)	Establish dietary prescription in collaboration with a dietitian.
	Prescribe dietary supplement (to be taken 1 to 2 hours after meals). *Several small meals and snacks are less fatiguing than are three large meals.*
Consume a well-balanced, high-calorie diet (2400 calories as evidenced by the following:	
Establishes a pattern of 4 to 6 small meals per day after rest periods	Teach and monitor use of food diary (include family member and patient). *Documenting oral intake and patient's progress facilitates early detection of inadequate intake.*
Uses bronchodilators and steroids with food/milk products	
Gradually increases dietary supplement from 2 to 6 oz twice a day	Help patient to identify food preferences, including foods high in complex carbohydrates and high in protein.
Reports less gastric distress	

---

*For the patient with chronic obstructive lung disease.

continued.

Nutrition, Altered: Less Than Body Requirements—cont'd

PATIENT GOALS/ EXPECTED OUTCOMES	NURSING INTERVENTIONS/ *SCIENTIFIC RATIONALE*
	Assist family member in planning high-calorie, high-protein meals. *Several small additions, such as adding margarine or butter to hot cereal, will greatly increase the calorie intake.* Encourage family member to avoid overemphasizing diet. Teach importance of oral hygiene before meals *to enhance taste.*
Establish a pattern of rest/ activity that enables participation in desired activities as evidenced by the following:	
Rests 1 hour before and after meals Paces ADLs Does active ROM exercises twice a day Uses portable oxygen to gradually increase walking distance by 5-ft increments	Teach pacing of ADLs. Instruct patient/family member in use of energy conservation techniques. Teach appropriate use of oxygen to increase ability to engage in exercise. *Independence in self-care will maximize the patient's self-esteem and compliance.*
Practices inspiratory muscle-training exercises as scheduled Establishes a regular bedtime routine Avoids use of stimulating beverages Enrolls in out-patient pulmonary rehabilitation program Engages in outside social activity weekly	Teach/monitor inspiratory muscle-training exercises. *Increasing inspiratory muscle strength may help reduce shortness of breath.* Teach patient self-care practices to prevent respiratory infection. If bronchitis develops, consult physician for antibiotic prescription as appropriate. *Infection increases the work of breathing.*

Nutrition, Altered: Less Than Body Requirements—cont'd

PATIENT GOALS/ EXPECTED OUTCOMES	NURSING INTERVENTIONS/ SCIENTIFIC RATIONALE
	Teach patient/family member use of exercise log to record distance walked, use of oxygen supplement, and feelings of breathlessness. *Nutritional support needs to be accompanied and supported by conditioning exercises.*

References 46, 245, 525, 610a.

Related factors: Long-established eating habits; no regular pattern of exercise

Colleen O'Brien, Marie Maguire, and Audrey M. McLane

PATIENT GOALS/ EXPECTED OUTCOMES	NURSING INTERVENTIONS/ SCIENTIFIC RATIONALE
Achieve gradual weight loss to 5% to 10% over ideal weight as evidenced by the following: Loses 1 to 2 lb per week Rewards self for each 5-lb weight loss	Help patient identify importance of weight loss. Explore motivation to lose weight; reinforce if necessary. Reinforce commitment to lose weight. *Motivation occurs when the patient identifies significant need.* Monitor weight weekly *to provide feedback/reinforcement.*
Eat a well-balanced diet as evidenced by the following: Keeps a daily food diary Chooses foods from the food pyramid groups Decreases intake of sweets from daily, to every other day, to twice a week	Teach use of food diary *to facilitate self-monitoring.* Analyze (with patient) food diary weekly (include food eaten, time of day, surroundings, circumstances, where eating occurs). Suggest techniques to change eating behaviors. Identify low-calorie food preferences. *Identifying food preferences increases likelihood of compliance.* Make recommendations for dietary changes in collaboration with patient. Encourage water consumption to 8 glasses a day, *which will provide adequate hydration necessary for body's metabolism.*

Nutrition, Altered: More Than Body Requirements—cont'd

PATIENT GOALS/ EXPECTED OUTCOMES	NURSING INTERVENTIONS/ *SCIENTIFIC RATIONALE*
	Teach use of cognitive coping strategies (e.g., distraction, thought stopping). *Variety of strategies may increase success.* Establish written contract with patient to use techniques to modify eating behaviors.
Participate in regular exercise as evidenced by the following:	
Engages in regular exercise for 20 minutes 3 times a week	Offer pamphlets/samples of exercises for the elderly. Explore option of taking daily walks. *Exercise increases the calories expended and facilitates weight loss.*
Keeps an exercise log	Explain/review use of exercise log. Help patient to develop a pattern of nonfood rewards for each 5-lb weight loss. *Exercise log and rewards reinforce positive behavior and promote motivation.* Establish written contract with patient to increase activity level. *Contracts validate commitment.*

References 80, 374, 491, 548, 556, 628.

Nutrition, Altered: High Risk for More Than Body Requirements

Risk factors: Disruption of relationship with significant other; dysfunctional pattern of intake

Jane Lancour and Audrey M. McLane

PATIENT GOALS/ EXPECTED OUTCOMES	NURSING INTERVENTIONS/ *SCIENTIFIC RATIONALE*
Alter pattern of intake as evidenced by the following:	
Holds present weight for 1 week followed by loss of 1 to 2 lb per week until desired weight is achieved	Develop a method for patient to keep a daily record of intake and cues associated with intake.
Verbalizes the relationship between experience of loss and pattern of intake	Analyze log weekly to determine relationship of patient's feelings to pattern of intake.
	Identify with patient desired weight.
	Determine desirable weekly loss.
	Develop with patient a diet prescription.
	Evaluate intake patterns for balance in major food groups.
Limits alcohol intake to one drink, containing no more than 1 oz of alcohol, per week	Alert patient to dangers of using alcohol as a coping strategy.
Increase energy expenditure as evidenced by the following:	
Translates awareness of need for increased physical activity into energy utilization tactics (e.g., uses stairs, walks to grocery store)	Help patient to identify, select, and participate in one or more energy-expending activities.
Schedules/participates in energy-expending diversional activities for 30 minutes daily	Monitor involvement in selected activity(ies).
	Patients need help incorporating exercise into their daily lives. Planning to exercise three times a week is more difficult to implement than exercising daily, i.e., making a life-style change.

Nutrition, Altered: High Risk for More Than Body Requirements—cont'd

PATIENT GOALS/ EXPECTED OUTCOMES	NURSING INTERVENTIONS/ SCIENTIFIC RATIONALE
Engage in relationships/activities that facilitate positive coping as evidenced by the following: Seeks support and assistance from selected relationships	Assist patient in identifying pattern of social relationships using social network tool. Help patient to verbalize his/her responses to efforts to increase/strengthen social network. Maintain an atmosphere of genuineness, empathy, and unconditional positive regard. Monitor influence of social interaction on food intake.

References 7, 17a, 55, 71a, 130, 319a, 595a.

Oral Mucous Membrane, Altered

ORAL MUCOUS MEMBRANE, ALTERED

Related factor: Trauma associated with chemotherapy
Rosemarie Suhayda and Mi Ja Kim

PATIENT GOALS/ EXPECTED OUTCOMES	NURSING INTERVENTIONS/ SCIENTIFIC RATIONALE
Maintain a comfortable and functional oral cavity as evidenced by the following: Pink, moist, and intact mucosa, tongue, and lips Absence of inflammation, lesions, crusts, or hard debris. Absence of infection Feeling of oral cleanliness Comfort in swallowing and talking	Establish a mouth care regimen before and after meals and at bedtime *to prevent infection.* For severe stomatitis, increase mouth care to every 2 hours and twice at night. *Omission of oral hygiene for periods of 2 to 6 hours nullifies past benefits of care.* Remove dentures. Brush, soak, and cleanse thoroughly. In case of severe stomatitis instruct patient to remove dentures for periods of time. *Dentures will irritate inflamed mucosa and cause necrotic ulceration, bleeding, pain when eating or talking.* Select a powerful spray or small, soft toothbrush for removal of dental debris. To soften toothbrush, soak in hot water before brushing, and rinse in hot water during brushing. Rinse well after use and store in cool dry place. *Toothbrushes may be contraindicated in severe stomatitis, thrombocytopenia, and neutropenia.* Use a finger wrapped in gauze to help remove dental debris.

Oral Mucous Membrane, Altered—cont'd

PATIENT GOALS/ EXPECTED OUTCOMES	NURSING INTERVENTIONS/ *SCIENTIFIC RATIONALE*
	Use toothettes or disposable foam swabs *to stimulate gums and clean oral cavity.* Avoid use of lemon-glycerine swabs, *which irritate the oral mucosa and contribute to tooth decalcification.* Encourage flossing between teeth twice a day with unwaxed dental floss if platelet levels are above 50,000/mm. Encourage frequent rinsing of mouth with mouthwashes and gargles *to cleanse the mouth, reduce microscopic flora, and soothe and relieve local discomfort.* Either of the following may be used: Sodium bicarbonate solution: 7 oz H_2O, ½ tsp salt, ½ tsp sodium bicarbonate. Discard unused mouthwash every 2 days (may have an unpleasant taste and be irritating). *Sodium bicarbonate helps remove thick mucus.* Warm saline (frequently solution of choice; may not be effective in removing hardened crusts or debris.) *Warm saline is a nonirritating and efficient way to apply heat to inflamed mucus membranes.*

continued.

Oral Mucous Membrane, Altered—cont'd

PATIENT GOALS/ EXPECTED OUTCOMES	NURSING INTERVENTIONS/ *SCIENTIFIC RATIONALE*
	Use an oxidizing agent such as hydrogen peroxide in a quarter-strength or 1.5% commercially available solution. Avoid prolonged use, *because such use can cause fungal growth called "hairy tongue." Hydrogen peroxide exerts an effervescent action that mechanically removes debris.*

References 35, 66, 138-140, 550.

Pain (Acute)

Related factors: Inadequate pain relief from prn. analgesic; reluctance to take pain medication*

Audrey M. McLane

PATIENT GOALS/ EXPECTED OUTCOMES	NURSING INTERVENTIONS/ *SCIENTIFIC RATIONALE*
Obtain pain relief as evidenced by the following:	
Verbalizes comfort and pain relief after analgetic is administered	Administer narcotic analgetic as appropriate
Reports 3 to 4 hours of uninterrupted sleep at night	Use a flow sheet to monitor pain in terms of quality, intensity, duration, effects of narcotic(s), and comfort measures *to determine adequacy of pain medication.*
Alternates periods of activity/ rest	Collaborate with physician to establish a regular schedule for administration of parenteral/oral narcotics.
	Collaborate with physician to provide upward adjustment of dose when substituting oral for parenteral narcotic.
	Teach patient/significant other to continue scheduled narcotic use at home to maximize pain relief.
	Provide patient/significant other with verbal/written, accurate information about narcotic analgetics.
	Teach patient/significant other that taking pain medication is appropriate.
	Assist patient/significant other with downward adjustment of narcotic (if indicated) after discharge/completion of chemotherapy.

*For the patient 2 days after surgery for inoperable cancer.   *continued.*

Pain (Acute)—cont'd

PATIENT GOALS/ EXPECTED OUTCOMES	NURSING INTERVENTIONS/ *SCIENTIFIC RATIONALE*
	Collaboration with physician and patient/significant other provides opportunity for joint evaluation of analgetic regimen.
Augment narcotic-induced pain relief as evidenced by the following: Uses music tapes, TV, and radio for diversion Learns/uses progressive muscle relaxation Collaborates with nurse to test/evaluate selected cognitive strategies and physical measures to augment comfort and pain control	Provide information about various strategies to augment pain relief (relaxation, guided imagery, diversional activities, and so on). Teach/monitor patient use of selected strategies to augment pain relief. Test/evaluate use of physical measures, massage, heat, and so on, to increase patient comfort. Teach patient/significant other to use daily log of pain and activities to determine what precipitates/relieves pain. *Diversion through use of auditory stimulation (e.g., music) may augment pain relief by release of endorphins.*
Maintain quality of life, hope, and faith as evidenced by the following: Increases participation in ADLs gradually by planning and pacing activities Makes fewer statements about fear of drug dependence	Teach family members ways to assist with ADLs. Teach patient/family to plan/pace ADLs. Provide positive feedback for small gains in self-care.

Pain (Acute)—cont'd

PATIENT GOALS/ EXPECTED OUTCOMES	NURSING INTERVENTIONS/ *SCIENTIFIC RATIONALE*
	Teach family members to use back massage and other comfort-inducing measures. *Use of comfort measures (e.g. back rub, clean sheets) may facilitate restful night's sleep and increase ability to cope with pain.*
	Enable patient/family to make decision about chemotherapy.
Plans with family/health team members for discharge, outpatient follow-up, and home care	Discuss with patient/family when/how to contact nurse/physician to assist with problem solving after discharge.
	Assist patient with values clarification and realistic goal setting.

References 112, 391, 516, 559, 572, 595.

PAIN, CHRONIC

Related factors: Inadequate knowledge of pain management*
Audrey M. McLane

PATIENT GOALS/ EXPECTED OUTCOMES	NURSING INTERVENTIONS/ *SCIENTIFIC RATIONALE*
Take an active role in pain management as evidenced by the following:	
Identifies measures that have helped relieve pain in the past	Elicit patient's ideas about measures to control pain.
Verbalizes desire to gain control over pain	Pay attention to language used to describe pain and its severity.
	Teach early intervention in the pain experience.
Records pain episodes, measures used to control pain, and pain relief	Teach/monitor use of pain log to record type of pain, measures used to control pain, and pain relief obtained. *Recording pain experiences and measures used to relieve pain increases patient's perception of control.*
Use a variety of pain control measures as evidenced by the following:	
Expresses willingness to try new strategies to augment pain relief	Elicit patient's knowledge of analgetics and nonsteroidal antiinflammatory drugs (NSAIDs) used to control pain.
Records relaxation practice sessions in pain log	Teach/coach/monitor relaxation techniques.
	Discuss importance of trying a pain-control technique more than one time. *Pain relief obtained from a pain control measure may differ from day to day; measure may not be effective the first time used.*

*For patient with chronic back pain, 2 months after laminectomy.

Pain, Chronic—cont'd

PATIENT GOALS/ EXPECTED OUTCOMES	NURSING INTERVENTIONS/ *SCIENTIFIC RATIONALE*
Uses heat and rest to augment pain relief	Instruct in safe use of heating pad; use moist heat (Thermophore). *Moist heat helps to relieve pain and promotes relaxation/rest.*

References 57, 195, 269, 359, 388, 521, 620, 624.

Related factor: Home care of a child with special technologic needs*

Donna M. Dixon, Karen Kavanaugh, Alice M. Tse, and Mi Ja Kim

PATIENT GOALS/ EXPECTED OUTCOMES	NURSING INTERVENTIONS/ SCIENTIFIC RATIONALE
Participate in technology-related care as evidenced by the following:	
Maintains desired levels of participation with health professionals	Monitor parents' desired level of participation in care and decision making. Provide consistent contact with health professionals for information gathering and follow-up.
Participates in routine and complex caretaking activities	Determine style of parental relationship with health professionals: limited contact, recipients of care, monitors of care, and managers of care *because parental participation differs according to the level of trust in professionals, information-gathering style, and decision-making patterns.*
Makes independent, safe decisions related to acute episodes of the illness, equipment malfunction, or need for professional assistance	Monitor knowledge base and competency related to equipment and required care. Assess level of anxiety related to skill performance.
Adapts information for the development of a personal style of performing skills.	Teach equipment operation, maintenance, safety, and necessary back-up. Teach CPR as necessary. Provide opportunities to master required home health-care skills when the child is hospitalized.

*For the family caring for children who require ventilators, tracheostomies, intravenous hyperalimentation, central venous catheters, apnea monitoring, and/or gastrostomy feedings.

Parental Role Conflict—cont'd

PATIENT GOALS/ EXPECTED OUTCOMES	NURSING INTERVENTIONS/ *SCIENTIFIC RATIONALE*
	Teach factors that increase frequency of complications, such as exposure to infections and immobility. Review management of acute episodes. Evaluate parents' understanding of special care and provide clarification as needed. *Learning is a complex process that requires time for integration into the family's current lifestyle. Continual assessment of barriers to learning, anxiety, and competency enhance the process.* Develop plans for ordering supplies and contacting vendors.
Express feelings and concerns about parental role demands as evidenced by the following: Verbalizes feelings and perceptions of self, role change, fears, and level of stress. Maintains roles of primary caretaker, educator, protector, and disciplinarian.	Monitor parents' perceptions of current situation as they compare with previous parenting patterns. Help parents to verbalize any fears, expectations for the future, feelings of isolation, and feelings of overwhelming responsibility. Determine extended family and friends' positive and negative reactions to child's situation. Assist the parents to involve the child in age-appropriate self-care and home responsibilities. Discuss ways to maintain appropriate parent-child relationship without overprotectiveness, guilt, or anger.

continued.

PARENTAL ROLE CONFLICT

PATIENT GOALS/ EXPECTED OUTCOMES	NURSING INTERVENTIONS/ *SCIENTIFIC RATIONALE*
Has adequate financial resources.	Assess financial status and concerns and refer to appropriate resources.
Has minimal health problems related to stress.	Counsel parents to develop strategies for the future to facilitate expression of feelings and concerns.
Maintains desired level of contact with significant others for emotional and caretaking support.	Refer to support groups and parents in similar situations as available and desired by the parents.
	Assess involvement in community religious groups.
	Teach patients about specific strategies used by families in difficult situations, such as acquiring social support, reframing, seeking spiritual support, mobilizing of family to acquire and accept support and passive appraisal. *Families of technology-assisted children often lack financial resources, feel isolated, receive unwanted advice from others, and expend tremendous energy mobilizing community assistance and support*
Incorporate technology in family life as evidenced by the following:	
Evaluates family boundaries, goals, patterns of interaction, and values in relation to the health of the child.	Assist family to identify stressors and strains related to incorporation of the technology, specific strengths related to the stage of development/career, and resources and capabilities related to their stage of development/career. *Long-term effects of pediatric home care vary over time and warrant continual reevaluation.*

Parental Role Conflict—cont'd

PATIENT GOALS/ EXPECTED OUTCOMES	NURSING INTERVENTIONS/ *SCIENTIFIC RATIONALE*
Develops adjustment strategies and problem-solving and adaptive coping skills.	Assist family to determine their accord about competencies as a family, such as quality of marital communication, shared orientation to childrearing and illness management, and satisfaction with quality of life. *Adaptability is the ability of the family to reorganize its power structure, roles, and rules. Emotional bonding, boundaries, supports, and time for recreation influence family cohesion.*
Integrates new patterns of behavior and responsibility into individual, family, and school routines.	Help parents incorporate necessary life-style changes. Provide anticipatory guidance about schooling and/or child care. Help family to plan and implement necessary social and environmental adaptions at home and school. Assist parents to involve siblings in the care of the child and home responsibilities. Assist parents to involve the child in age-appropriate self-care and home responsibilities. *A family management style develops when a family incorporates the care of a chronically ill child.*

References 18, 113, 196, 298, 299, 441, 458, 485, 518, 558, 566.

Parenting, Altered (Actual)

Related factors: Inadequate role identity; unrealistic expectations

Martha M. Morris and Gertrude K. McFarland

PATIENT GOALS/ EXPECTED OUTCOMES	NURSING INTERVENTIONS/ *SCIENTIFIC RATIONALE*
Provide safe environment for child as evidenced by the following: Child remains physically and psychologically safe	Assess the parents' awareness of the child's needs. Assess degree of risk to child's physical and psychological safety. Contact appropriate authorities if child's safety seems jeopardized. *Providing a physically and psychologically safe environment for the child is the basic function of a parent. Deficiencies in this area may range from routinely ignoring a child's diet or personal hygiene to homes with multiple safety hazards to severe physical abuse.* Design specific interventions to focus the parents' awareness of the child's needs. *In situations where the parent cannot provide for the minimal safety and physiological needs of the child, mechanisms designed by the community must be engaged to remove the child to a safer envionment.*

Parenting, Altered (Actual)—cont'd

PATIENT GOALS/ EXPECTED OUTCOMES	NURSING INTERVENTIONS/ SCIENTIFIC RATIONALE
Achieve role identity as parent as evidenced by the following:	
Identifies socially expected parenting behaviors	Identify major components and priorities within role identity (i.e., child of one's parents, spouse, professional identity).
Verbalizes presence or absence of effective role models	
Verbalizes incongruency between "ideal" parenting behaviors and actual behaviors.	Identify source of verbalized "ideal" parenting behavior.
	Identify perception of specific parenting behaviors.
Incorporates concept of "parent" as integral part of role identity	Observe parent-child interactions for congruency between verbalized "ideal" of parent behavior and actual behavior.
Demonstrates learning of additional parenting behavior	Provide opportunity for parent to explore role identity through individual counseling and/or group interaction.
	Provide opportunity for parent to observe/experience effective parenting behaviors. *Parenting is a learned behavior. In many communities the opportunity for observing parenting behavior is limited, and persons are forced to rely on their perception of how they were parented.*
Experiences satisfaction in parenting that will support incorporation of concept of "parent" into role identity	Provide opportunity for parent to implement alternative parenting behaviors. *Interventions that provide information about alternative parenting behaviors and opportunity to discuss the changes in life-style required broaden the parent's perspective and aid in internalizing the parenting role.*

continued.

PARENTING, ALTERED (ACTUAL)

PATIENT GOALS/ EXPECTED OUTCOMES	NURSING INTERVENTIONS/ *SCIENTIFIC RATIONALE*
Acquire realistic expectations of self, spouse, and infant/child within family as evidenced by the following:	
Verbalizes expectations of self, spouse, and infant/child	Identify present expectations of self, spouse, and infant/child.
Verbalizes areas of failure to meet expectations	Identify areas of failure to meet self-expectations.
Verbalizes own feelings about expectations	Provide opportunity for parent to express feelings about unmet expectations.
Acknowledges own responsibility for attempting to meet expectations and realistic limits of self and others	Encourage parent to speculate on reasons for expectations being unmet.
Develop realistic expectations of self, spouse, and infant/child	Help parent to develop realistic expectations as result of increased knowledge of normal development and basic needs.
Develop strategies that increase the possibility that expectations will be met	Help parent to develop alternative strategies to increase possibility of having expectations met (e.g., discussing expectations with spouse, identifying steps that must occur to meet expectations.
	Parents may have unrealistic expectations of their role and abilities as a parent, of their spouse's role and abilities, and the child's role and ability in the relationship. These expectations may lead to increased frustration and anxiety as the expected behaviors are not manifested. Because anxiety is frequently transformed into anger, the potential for disruption of parenting function is great.

Parenting, Altered (Actual)—cont'd

PATIENT GOALS/ EXPECTED OUTCOMES	NURSING INTERVENTIONS/ *SCIENTIFIC RATIONALE*
	Help the parent to identify the source of the anger and develop more realistic expectations *to diffuse the anxiety and offer an opportunity to develop alternative behaviors*.

References 51, 98, 228, 261, 263, 299, 440.

Parenting, Altered High Risk for

PARENTING, ALTERED HIGH RISK FOR

Risk factors: Inadequate knowledge

Martha M. Morris and Gertrude K. McFarland

PATIENT GOALS/ EXPECTED OUTCOMES	NURSING INTERVENTIONS/ SCIENTIFIC RATIONALE
Acquire adequate knowledge base for effective parenting as evidenced by the following:	
Verbalizes desired knowledge about specific aspects of parenting	Identify knowledge deficits.
	Identify learning readiness and learning capability of parent.
Demonstrates more effective parenting behavior, such as consistent discipline and providing for child's physical, psychological, emotional, and social needs	Provide opportunity for parent to test out new information.
	Encourage play activities between parent and child.
	Encourage age-appropriate caretaking activities by parents.
	Create a positive learning environment.
	Lack of information, role models, and external resources and ineffective coping skills may all be decreased through appropriate patient education methods.
Experience emotional, social, and physical support for optimal parenting role as evidenced by the following:	
Recognizes realistic limitations of self and support systems	Identify specific areas of needed emotional, social, and/or physical support. *Many of the defining characteristics of Altered Parenting are the result of insufficient emotional, social, or physical support.*

PATIENT GOALS/ EXPECTED OUTCOMES	NURSING INTERVENTIONS/ SCIENTIFIC RATIONALE
Selects appropriate resources to supplement self and support system	Identify specific strengths of parent and support systems. Encourage parent to express feelings about areas of need. *Persons whose own basic needs for safety, nutrition, or love have not been met will be unable to meet the needs of another.*
Learns to activate additional support systems as needed	Provide information about additional resources available to meet areas of need. *Once specific areas of deficiencies have been identified, the nurse may offer information about services available to provide the support needed.* Act as liaison/advocate as needed in obtaining help from appropriate resources.

References 16, 33, 234, 261, 538, 540, 612.

Peripheral Neurovascular Dysfunction, High Risk for

Risk factors: Mechanical compression
Joyce Johnson and Mi Ja Kim

PATIENT GOALS/ EXPECTED OUTCOMES	NURSING INTERVENTIONS/ *SCIENTIFIC RATIONALE*
Maintain neurovascular integrity to the extremity as evidenced by the following: Has absence of pain, pallor or cyanosis, pulselessness, paraesthesia, and paralysis ("five Ps") Progresses through cast, splint, or brace therapy without experiencing complications Notifies nurse/physician of signs and symptoms of peripheral neurovascular compromise while in the hospital and after discharge	Perform neurovascular assessment every hour for first 24 hours; then every 2 hours for 8 hours; then every 4 hours. Continue as long as mechanical compression is present (extremity cast, check involved distal extremity; spica or body cast, check all four extremities; halo cast, check cranial nerves). Observe capillary filling after compression of arteries of extremity. *Failure of circulatory return to extremity when pressure is released indicates arterial injury.* Feel temperature of both extremities. Observe color of skin. Observe for presence and amount of edema (e.g., insert fingers under cast or measure circumference of extremities. *As swelling within muscle compartment increases, neurovascular compromise occurs.* Palpate pulses. Monitor for evidence of paraesthesia and decreased or absence of sensation, including 2-point discrimination. *2-point discrimination is the best check of sensitivity.*

Peripheral Neurovascular Dysfunction, High Risk for – cont'd

PATIENT GOALS/ EXPECTED OUTCOMES	NURSING INTERVENTIONS/ SCIENTIFIC RATIONALE
	Assess mobility (flexion, extension, abduction, and adduction) of fingers and toes. Bring tips of thumb and fingers together to form circle. *Performing circle maneuver is impossible if radial, ulnar, and median nerves are not intact to intrinsic muscles.*
	Assess for pain out of proportion to injury. *The primary concern of neurovascular dysfunction is impairment of nerves or blood vessels distal to the area of the cast, splint, or traction. Early detection of neurovascular compromise can avoid irreversible and permanent damage.*
	Document and report immediately any evidence of neurovascular compromise. *Permanent and irreversible damage resulting in paresis, paralysis, or amputation can occur rapidly, even over a period of hours.*
	Elevate extremity to level of heart until edema is controlled.
	Avoid elevating extremity above person's central venous pressure (CVP); normal CVP = 6-13 cm H_2O pressure; 2.5 cm = 1 inch.

continued.

PATIENT GOALS/ EXPECTED OUTCOMES	NURSING INTERVENTIONS/ SCIENTIFIC RATIONALE
	Elevating extremity aids venous return to decrease edema. Elevating extremity above person's CVP impedes arterial flow and increases edema rather than decreases it.
	Apply icebags to lateral surfaces of cast or traction for 24 to 48 hours—avoid placing over arterial areas. *Cold decreases edema; applying over artery could impede arterial flow.*
	Avoid pressure over peroneal nerve.
	Observe for paresthesia of anterior surface of affected leg, dorsum of foot and great toe, and inability to dorsiflex foot/extend toes. *Pressure on peroneal nerve can result in permanent foot drop.*
	Split cast down one or both sides and rewrap split cast with elastic bandage, if necessary; remove traction/splint and reapply more loosely. *Irreversible and permanent damage can result in 6 hours if pressure is not relieved.*
	Instruct patient/significant other about signs and symptoms of peripheral neurovascular compromise.

Peripheral Neurovascular Dysfunction, High Risk for — cont'd

PATIENT GOALS/ EXPECTED OUTCOMES	NURSING INTERVENTIONS/ *SCIENTIFIC RATIONALE*
	Emphasize importance of notifying nurse/physician immediately of numbness or tingling, increasing pain, increased swelling, or change in color. *Complications from cast, splint, or traction therapy can occur at any time. Changes in weight, edema loss, and softening of the cast can create changes in neurovascular status.*
Prevent compartment syndrome and Volkmann's ischemic fracture resulting from compression or severance of an artery as evidenced by the following:	
Normal compartment pressure (<10 mm Hg)	Assess for increasing and progressive pain on passive motion. *Pain on passive motion is the earliest and most significant sign of compartment syndrome.*
Adequate tissue perfusion, as noted by brisk (<3 sec) capillary refill	
Normal ROM in all extremities	Assess for evidence of pallor or cyanosis. *Tissue damage results when oxygen is reduced because of lack of blood supply; hypoxia resulting from entrapment of vessels or nerves can result in ischemic contracture or ischemic myositis.*
	Immobilize traumatized extremity. *Movement of arm or leg can result in further injury to nerves and blood vessels.*

continued.

Peripheral Neurovascular Dysfunction, High Risk for– cont'd

PATIENT GOALS/ EXPECTED OUTCOMES	NURSING INTERVENTIONS/ *SCIENTIFIC RATIONALE*
	Perform and document tissue pressure readings. *Normal tissue pressure is 0 to 10 mm Hg. Increase in pressure denotes impending compartment syndrome.*
	Immediately report tissue pressure readings of 30 mm Hg or above. *Pressures of 30 mm Hg or above can result in irreversible damage if not relieved within 6 hours; 30 mm Hg is the criterion used for surgical decompression. If pressure in the compartment equals diastolic blood pressure, microcirculation ceases.*

References 94, 167, 206, 246, 367, 409, 443, 448, 472.

Personal Identity Disturbance

Related factors: History of severe, traumatic interpersonal experiences; multiple current stressors*

Gertrude K. McFarland and Karen E. Inaba

PATIENT GOALS/ EXPECTED OUTCOMES	NURSING INTERVENTIONS/ SCIENTIFIC RATIONALE
Maintain positive concept of personal identity as evidenced by the following: Demonstrates positive acceptance and identification of self Identifies self with a sense of continuity over time	Develop trusting relationship with patient with ongoing dialogue about safety and trust. Review patient's values, beliefs, and goals *to assess sense of self and self-awareness.* Encourage patient to verbalize about relationships and experiences that have influenced self-concept *to determine impact of past severe traumatic interpersonal experiences and possible sources of anxiety or pain.* Support positive self-designations and self-affirmation statements *to reinforce positive self-image and competencies.* Encourage independent decision making, providing nonjudgmental feedback. Use role playing and role reversal to try out new behaviors *to decrease anxiety and support problem-solving.* Mobilize social support from significant others.

*For the patient with borderline personality disorder.

continued.

PERSONAL IDENTITY DISTURBANCE

PATIENT GOALS/ EXPECTED OUTCOMES	NURSING INTERVENTIONS/ *SCIENTIFIC RATIONALE*
Distinguish between self and nonself as evidenced by the following:	
Perceives and responds to others as separate from self	Set limits around personal boundaries and clarify expectations about the nurse-patient relationship *to decrease ambivalence and anxiety.*
Integrates thoughts, emotions, and behavior into an organized self	Modify environmental stressors *to decrease a sense of threat and disorganization.*
	Support patient's independence *to help reinforce separateness and differentiation.*
	Teach patient stress-management techniques.
	Monitor mental status *to identify presence of organic causes of symptoms and reality-testing difficulties.*

References 28, 79, 97, 185, 191, 325, 356, 496, 513, 524.

Poisoning, High Risk for

Risk factors: Large stock of medications stored in an inappropriate place; poor lighting*

Audrey M. McLane

PATIENT GOALS/ EXPECTED OUTCOMES	NURSING INTERVENTIONS/ *SCIENTIFIC RATIONALE*
Adapt home environment to reduce risk of accidental poisoning as evidenced by the following:	
Selects an appropriate storage area for medications	Collaborate with patient to establish separate storage area for medications.
Permanently removes all cleaning supplies from bathroom	Evaluate (with patient) contents of medicine cabinet and discard outdated medications.
Discards outdated drugs	
Replaces 25- and 60-watt bulbs with larger bulbs where appropriate	Teach patient to keep environment well lighted.
Keeps hall and bathroom lights on during evening and night	Teach patient to keep flashlight at bedside in case of power failure.
	Place list of emergency telephone numbers near telephone.
Establish/adhere to a safe method for taking medications as evidenced by the following:	
Uses magnifying glass to check contents of each bottle	Help patient to develop a way to identify medications accurately.
Sets up medications for 24-hour period in well-lighted area	Discuss and demonstrate way to set up medications for 24 hours. *Setting up medications for 24-hour period decreases risk of missing a dose or taking extra dose.*
Demonstrates agreed-on method to set up medications	
Counts with nurse amount of medication remaining in containers	Monitor medication taking.

*For the patient with reduced vision from cataracts in both eyes. *continued.*

PATIENT GOALS/ EXPECTED OUTCOMES	NURSING INTERVENTIONS/ SCIENTIFIC RATIONALE
Seek medical evaluation of reduced vision as evidenced by the following:	
Schedules an appointment for visit from social worker	Provide patient with list of medical and financial resources in community.
Makes/keeps appointment to see ophthalmologist	Help patient to make appointment.
Family members agree to assist with transportation to keep appointments	Develop plan with patient and family for medical evaluation.

References 187, 421, 460, 577.

Post-Trauma Response

Related factors: Temporary loss of mobility with fractures; overwhelming feelings of guilt/responsibility for auto accident
Audrey M. McLane

PATIENT GOALS/ EXPECTED OUTCOMES	NURSING INTERVENTIONS/ *SCIENTIFIC RATIONALE*
Develop/use new coping strategies to deal with excessive feelings of guilt as evidenced by the following:	
Reports 2 to 3 hours of uninterrupted sleep at night	Explore guilt feelings with patient relative to state of readiness *to provide an environment for free expression of feelings.*
	Identify strategies that patient has used in the past to induce sleep.
Decreases excessive verbalization of details of accident	Provide consultation/referral to deal with excessive feelings of guilt.
Maintains relationship with significant other	Contact family of significant other to obtain information about health status of significant other.
	Arrange for telephone visits/ personal visits with significant other.
	Allow for privacy during interactions with significant other.
Schedules regular visits with minister/pastor	Arrange for spiritual counseling (with patient's approval to contact minister/pastor).
Requests family members to maintain outside job and social obligations	Discuss with family members the need to fulfill outside obligations to avoid adding to patient's feelings of guilt.
Maintain relationships with loved ones and friends as evidenced by the following:	
Accepts assistance of parents and siblings to deal with outside obligations	Provide family members with information about patient's physical status.

continued.

Post-Trauma Response—cont'd

PATIENT GOALS/ EXPECTED OUTCOMES	NURSING INTERVENTIONS/ *SCIENTIFIC RATIONALE*
Asks parents to manage insurance/legal aspects of accident Requests visits from spiritual advisor Initiates telephone visits with friends and personal visits with close friends	Instruct family about importance of frequent, short visits from family members and close friends. Request family members to bring meaningful personal items for patient's use. Ask family members to prepare list of telephone numbers of friends/family for easy access. Discuss with family an interim interaction approach: answer patient's questions about accident but avoid excessive details, including pictures. *These actions help patient, family, and significant other to express and accept feelings and reactions to traumatic event.*
Maintain structural/physiological integrity of body systems as evidenced by the following: Retains muscle strength in unaffected limbs Retains full ROM in affected limbs Skin remains intact (no redness, abrasions, and so on) Circulation, sensory, and motor functions remain intact in affected limbs	Instruct and assist with active ROM in unaffected limbs. Assist with passive ROM in affected limbs (within limits imposed by injury). Make small changes in body position every 2 hours. Monitor/massage pressure-prone areas of skin. *Providing ROM and proper position assists in maintaining structural integrity of body systems.* Monitor warmth, sensation, and movement of fingers and toes in casted extremities.

Post-Trauma Response—cont'd

PATIENT GOALS/ EXPECTED OUTCOMES	NURSING INTERVENTIONS/ *SCIENTIFIC RATIONALE*
Maintains pretrauma pattern of urine and bowel elimination	Monitor adequate fluid and fiber intake to prevent bladder and bowel elimination problems. Provide for adequate intake of fluids and foods high in fiber.
Use assistive devices to enhance self-care ability as evidenced by the following:	
Transfers from bed to wheelchair with assistance of one person	Guide patient in learning transfer techniques.
Attends physical therapy sessions twice a day to gain muscle strength and learn crutch walking	Arrange for physical therapy twice a day to learn crutch walking.
Practices crutch walking with nursing assistance	Praise patient for small gains in managing ADLs.
Resumes responsibility for ADLs gradually within limits of injuries	Monitor for side effects of increased activity (e.g., increased discomfort/pain in affected limbs). *Focus on taking more responsibility for ADLs helps patient to control intrusive thoughts about accident.*

References 44, 67, 286, 389, 578.

POWERLESSNESS

Powerlessness

Related factors: Controlling/authoritative health-care environment; life-style of helplessness

Gertrude K. McFarland and Mary E. Markert

PATIENT GOALS/ EXPECTED OUTCOMES	NURSING INTERVENTIONS/ SCIENTIFIC RATIONALE
Experience an increased sense of control over life situation and own activities as evidenced by the following:	
Verbalizes positive feelings about own ability to achieve a sense of power and control in patient role performance while in an authoritarian health-care environment	Explore with the patient personal preferences, needs, values, and attitudes; assist patient in appraising readiness to initiate and sustain health behaviors. *Involving the patient in planning care enhances the potential for mastery.*
Verbalizes acceptance of life situations over which patient does not have control	Provide opportunities for the patient to express feelings about self and illness; acknowledge and accept expressions of fear, anger, or lack of response to information or events as a manifestation of the patient's distress. *Verbalizing/exploring feelings increase understanding of individual coping styles/defense mechanisms.*
	Identify past/present coping behaviors that are positive and reinforce use. *Awareness of past successes enhances self-confidence.*
	Encourage patient to identify when feelings of powerlessness/loss of control began/occur in authoritative health-care environment. *Awareness increases understanding of stressors that trigger feelings of powerlessness.*

Powerlessness—cont'd

PATIENT GOALS/ EXPECTED OUTCOMES	NURSING INTERVENTIONS/ SCIENTIFIC RATIONALE
	Encourage patient to feel a sense of partnership with health-care team and help patient communicate effectively with other health team members.
	Encourage patient's interest and curiosity in differing aspects of care.
	Provide positive reinforcement for improvement.
	Encourage expression of positive emotions (hope, faith, will-to-live, sense of purpose).
	Addressing issues of self-esteem provides sense of appreciation for patient's dignity and realistic success.
Recover reversible impaired functioning and compensate for irreversible loss as evidenced by the following: Engages in problem-solving behaviors Identifies barriers to health-related change	Adjust caregiver practices and modify the plan of care to support patient's sense of control and involvement in decision making.
	Create/modify the environment to facilitate active participation in self-care.
	Provide for patient's privacy needs.
	Eliminate unpredictability by informing patient of scheduled tests/procedures.
	Help the patient anticipate sensory experiences that accompany procedures.
	Provide relevant learning materials.

continued.

POWERLESSNESS

PATIENT GOALS/ EXPECTED OUTCOMES	NURSING INTERVENTIONS/ SCIENTIFIC RATIONALE
	Support patient's efforts to increase resources (e.g., obtaining data about new technology).
	Alleviate physical discomfort that diminishes energy reserve.
Sets goals and tries alternative adaptive behaviors	Offer alternatives to routine ADLs (e.g., ADL schedule change, diversional activities, visiting hours, treatment times).
	Encourage involvement of significant others if patient desires.
Self-monitors health-related actions	Teach self-monitoring.
	Provide referrals to self-help groups, clergy, and other support systems as appropriate.

References 83, 125, 151, 179, 308, 398, 568, 579.

Protection, Altered

Related factors: Altered immune function secondary to biotherapy*

Kathleen C. Sheppard and Audrey M. McLane

PATIENT GOALS/ EXPECTED OUTCOMES	NURSING INTERVENTIONS/ *SCIENTIFIC RATIONALE*
Maintain protective defenses as evidenced by the following:	
Establishes a pattern of personal hygiene consistent with other demands of daily living	Teach strategies to promote personal and environmental cleanliness.
	Assist with daily shower and oral hygiene.
Patient/family incorporates safety measures to prevent infection, bleeding	Monitor vital signs every 4 hours.
	Teach/demonstrate safety precautions.
Patient/family incorporates safety measures	Reorient/assist during periods of confusion.
	Skin and mucous membranes are the frontline of defense, and cleanliness decreases exposure to microbes. Early report of abnormal vital signs (e.g., fever) can reduce complications. Injury from falls and trauma has a high risk of complications due to deficient protective mechanisms.
Restore protective defenses as evidenced by the following:	
Maintains normal body weight	Establish diet plan in collaboration with patient/dietitian.
Maintains hydration (fluid balance)	Weight patient daily.
	Offer small, frequent meals.
	Prescribe dietary supplement as needed.
	Encourage fluid intake.
	Monitor intake and output.

*For the patient with chronic myelogenous leukemia who is receiving biological response modifier therapy (e.g., interferon therapy). Biological response modifiers are biological or chemical agents produced by the body that augment, direct, and restore the body's immune function. *continued.*

PROTECTION, ALTERED

PATIENT GOALS/ EXPECTED OUTCOMES	NURSING INTERVENTIONS/ *SCIENTIFIC RATIONALE*
Incorporates period of rest before/after activities Symptoms resolve in response to therapy	Teach measures to conserve energy (e.g., pacing of ADLs). Provide comfort for symptoms (e.g., chills, fever, myalgias). *Nausea, vomiting, anorexia, diarrhea, and stomatitis are associated with biotherapy and have an impact on nutritional status and fluid balance. Fatigue is a component of biotherapy and is a dose-limiting toxicity. Flulike symptoms cause distress and may lead to stress and decreased quality of life.*
Promote protective defenses as evidenced by the following: Reports increased sense of well-being Incorporates new coping behaviors to deal with health challenge	Initiate stress management. Teach relaxation exercises. Teach alternate coping strategies. Assist with communication between patient and family. Provide nurse presence. *Psychoneuroimmunology provides rationale for mind-body interactions, stress, and immunodepression, and justifies interventions of touching, listening, and caring attitudes of the nurse.*

References 2, 75, 137, 220, 254, 444, 534, 535, 536, 603.

Rape-Trauma Syndrome: Acute Phase

Related factors: Fear of reprisal; anxiety about AIDS*
Audrey M. McLane and Pamela Kohlbry

PATIENT GOALS/ EXPECTED OUTCOMES	NURSING INTERVENTIONS/ SCIENTIFIC RATIONALE
Obtain relief from emotional responses to rape experience as evidenced by the following:	
Accepts immediate and ongoing counseling from rape-crisis center volunteer.	Acknowledge appropriateness of patient responses during/to victimization. Provide empathetic support during physician/police interveiws.
Identifies individual(s) in family/peer group who would provide support	Help patient identify individual(s) with whom rape experience could be discussed. *Women who receive crisis support recover more quickly than those who do not.*
Verbalizes decrease in fears, anxieties, and concerns	Assist staff/friends/family to focus on subjective experience of rape rather than on whether rape occurred. *A nonjudgmental attitude helps to allay/alleviate feelings of guilt/self-blame.*
Assume decision-making role as evidenced by the following:	
Asks questions that enable her to make decisions about health care	Offer information about medical/legal options to facilitate making choices. Identify decisions that can be postponed. *Rape challenges individual's sense of power, autonomy, and control; making own decisions can maintain power, sense of control, and feeling of responsibility.*

*For the patient who lives alone.

continued.

Rape-Trauma Syndrome: Acute Phase—cont'd

RAPE-TRAUMA SYNDROME: ACUTE PHASE

PATIENT GOALS/ EXPECTED OUTCOMES	NURSING INTERVENTIONS/ SCIENTIFIC RATIONALE
Makes appointment to discuss HIV testing and accepts written information about ethical issues surrounding HIV testing	Discuss benefit of periodic HIV testing, 5-year window of infection, and right to know assailant's HIV status vs. right to privacy and informed consent. Provide written information about ethical issues related to HIV testing and potential loss of employment/access to health insurance if seropositive. *Individual has the right to know benefits/risks of HIV testing and status of current debate about ethical/legal issues.*
Cope with concern for personal safety as evidenced by the following: Asks family member/peer to stay with her for a few days Sets goal of returning to usual activities by a specified date	Collaborate with patient to identify safety measures to decrease vulnerability. Provide a list of immediate and long-term responses to rape experience, (e.g., nightmares, flashbacks); emphasize reactions are not unusual.

References 85, 85a, 86, 320, 321, 358.

Rape-Trauma Syndrome: Compound Reaction

Related factors: Inadequate support system; inability to resolve rape-trauma experience compounded by current multiple stressors and previous traumatic experiences
Pamela Kohlbry and Audrey M. McLane

PATIENT GOALS/ EXPECTED OUTCOMES	NURSING INTERVENTIONS/ *SCIENTIFIC RATIONALE*
Develop significant other/ family support as evidenced by the following:	
Verbalizes that significant other has begun to express warmth and concern	Assist significant other/family to focus on subjective experi- ence of rape. Help patient identify individ- ual(s) with whom rape experi- ence could be discussed.
Accepts and keeps appointment with counselor at rape center	Refer patient/significant other to rape counseling center. Determine need for family to seek counseling. *Failure of significant other/fam- ily to provide support during the crisis period leads to feel- ings of guilt and self-blame; feelings require resolution be- fore current physical and emo- tional problems can be suc- cessfully treated.*
Make realistic decisions about actual/potential health problems as evi- denced by the following:	
Keeps follow-up medical ap- pointments	Teach importance of medication regimen.
Takes medication in keeping with prescribed regimen	Monitor adherence to medical regimen.
Makes appointment to discuss HIV testing and accepts writ- ten information about ethical issues surrounding HIV testing	Discuss benefit of periodic HIV testing, 5-year window of in- fection, and right to know as- sailant's HIV status vs. right of privacy and informed con- sent.

*For the patient who did not seek medical or psychological assistance at the time of rape.

continued.

Rape-Trauma Syndrome: Compound Reaction—cont'd

PATIENT GOALS/ EXPECTED OUTCOMES	NURSING INTERVENTIONS/ SCIENTIFIC RATIONALE
	Provide written information about ethical issues related to HIV testing and potential loss of employment/access to health insurance if seropositive.
	Individual has the right to know benefits/risks of HIV testing and status of current debate about ethical/legal issues.
Cope with cognitive and emotional responses to rape and other stressors as evidenced by the following:	
Verbalizes anger; resolves self-blame	Teach relaxation strategies. Monitor evolution/resolution of symptoms using Rape-Trauma Symptom Rating Scale.
Practices relaxation and cognitive coping strategies	Teach use of cognitive coping strategies: thought stopping, desensitization, guided imagery, refuting irrational ideas, and so on.
Participates in rape support group	Provide information about support group opportunities/benefits.
Significant other and patient keep/discuss feelings recorded in separate journals	Teach/monitor use of journal to express anger and related feelings.
	Discussing anger and related feelings enables couple to support one another.
	Provide/discuss written list of long-term responses to rape experience; emphasize reactions are not unusual.

Rape-Trauma Syndrome: Compound Reaction—cont'd

PATIENT GOALS/ EXPECTED OUTCOMES	NURSING INTERVENTIONS/ SCIENTIFIC RATIONALE
Resume a satisfying life-style as evidenced by the following:	
Reestablishes intimate relationship with spouse	Collaborate with patient in pacing social activities.
Reports feeling more secure	Identify/select strategies to protect from future assaults.
Maintains contact with legal system	Monitor/support patient's experiences with legal system.

References 85, 85a, 86, 153, 320, 321.

Rape-Trauma Syndrome: Silent Reaction

Related factors: Fear of retaliation; denial

Audrey M. McLane and Pamela Kohlbry

PATIENT GOALS/ EXPECTED OUTCOMES	NURSING INTERVENTIONS/ *SCIENTIFIC RATIONALE*
Cope with concern for personal safety as evidenced by the following:	
Verbalizes feelings of insecurity	Establish a trusting relationship with patient.
	Actively listen to patient's perceptions of increased vulnerability.
	Collaborate with patient to identify safety measures to decrease vulnerability.
Makes some progress in relating anxiety about safety to the rape event	Assist patient to identify source of anxiety about personal safety.
	Provide opportunity to discuss safety concerns with a female police officer.
	Focusing on establishing a trusting relationship and on providing direct assistance with safety measures may reduce fear enough to deal with unidentified problem of rape.
Decrease reliance on full denial to maintain sense of well-being as evidenced by the following:	
Begins to verbalize feeling of anger and shame related to rape	During routine interview, ask patient if anyone has ever attempted to assault her or hurt her in any way.
Verbalizes fear of male friends and relatives since rape	Avoid direct questioning; allow patient to continue at own pace to reveal details of own rape.
	Determine readiness for referral to rape counselor.

Rape-Trauma Syndrome: Silent Reaction—cont'd

PATIENT GOALS/ EXPECTED OUTCOMES	NURSING INTERVENTIONS/ SCIENTIFIC RATIONALE
Reveals some details of rape experience	Help patient identify specific concerns related to rape experience (e.g., concern about STDs and pregnancy).
Identifies individual in family who could provide support	Help patient identify one individual with whom rape experience could be discussed.
	Avoiding direct confrontation of denial may enable patient to begin to deal with fears/anxieties.
Assume decision-making role about health-care needs as evidenced by the following:	
Asks questions about health-care resources	Offer information about medical/legal options to facilitate making choices.
	Identify decisions that should be made soon and those which can be postponed.
Verbalizes fear of AIDS	Offer information about HIV testing. Discuss benefit of periodic HIV testing, 5-year window of infection, and right to know assailant's HIV status vs. right of privacy and informed consent.
Does not return to full denial during discussion of HIV testing	Provide written information about ethical issues related to HIV testing and potential loss of employment/access to health insurance if seropositive.
	Individual has the right to know benefits/risks of HIV testing and status of current debate about ethical/legal issues.

continued.

PATIENT GOALS/ EXPECTED OUTCOMES	NURSING INTERVENTIONS/ SCIENTIFIC RATIONALE
Cope with cognitive and emotional responses to rape experience as evidenced by the following:	
Verbalizes anger; resolves self-blame	Teach use of cognitive coping strategies (e.g., thought stopping, desensitization, guided imagery, refuting irrational ideas).
Practices cognitive coping strategies	Provide information about support group opportunities/benefits.
Participates in rape support group	Teach/monitor use of journal to express anger and related feelings.
	Discussion of fear, anger, and related feelings enables individual to obtain support from group.

References 85, 85a, 86, 153, 320, 321.

Relocation Stress Syndrome

Related factors: Sudden environmental change; recent migration*

Karen E. Inaba and Gertrude K. McFarland

PATIENT GOALS/ EXPECTED OUTCOMES	NURSING INTERVENTIONS/ SCIENTIFIC RATIONALE
Adapt to changes in environment as evidenced by the following:	
Demonstrates reduced levels of anxiety and grieving	Establish a supportive relationship with patient *to build trust and a sense of security.* Orient patient to new surroundings and routines *to decrease anxiety and sense of disruption.* Assess patient's current level of stressors (e.g., resettlement and acculturation stress, developmental crises, family roles, impact of changed health status) *to determine patient's perception of events and level of vulnerability.*
Identifies changes and losses associated with relocation (e.g., loss of culture, status, roles, social network)	Provide opportunities for patient to verbalize about perceived or actual changes and losses associated with relocation.
Maintains sense of self-worth and positive personal identity during transition to new setting	Acknowledge patient's cultural preferences whenever possible (e.g., diet, family involvement, communication patterns) and incorporate into care.
Makes positive statements about the new environment	Use consultants when appropriate (e.g., language translators, volunteers from culture-specific community programs) *to facilitate communication with patient.*
Expresses acceptance of changed surroundings and living arrangements	Protect patient's privacy and encourage autonomy and participation in decision making *to decrease powerlessness and feelings of marginality.*

*For an Indochinese immigrant patient with a pelvic fracture.

continued.

PATIENT GOALS/ EXPECTED OUTCOMES	NURSING INTERVENTIONS/ *SCIENTIFIC RATIONALE*
	Provide structure and consistent caregivers whenever possible *to minimize further changes for the patient and to foster continuity.* Assess sources of social support for patient (e.g., family, friends, ethnic community, religious organization) and facilitate contact.
Use help from appropriate resources during adjustment period to new environment as evidenced by the following:	
Initiates contact with health-care providers and community agencies Participates in support groups in current setting or community Establishes supportive personal relationships in new location	Initiate early discharge planning for culturally relevant follow-up in the community. Refer patient to self-help support groups (e.g., resettlement classes, church activities) to rebuild disrupted social network and *to promote feelings of universality and support during adjustment period.* Initiate early patient pretransfer teaching, working with language translators and others in patient's support system. Assess for any potential coping problems or inadequate support network and refer to mental health team.

References 27, 176, 295, 296, 322, 324, 368, 371, 480, 555.

Role Performance, Altered

Related factors: Situational transition, physical disability*
Gertrude K. McFarland and Karen E. Inaba

PATIENT GOALS/ EXPECTED OUTCOMES	NURSING INTERVENTIONS/ SCIENTIFIC RATIONALE
Engage in functional role performance as evidenced by the following:	
Specifies behaviors necessary for successful changed role expectations	Determine nature of role performance disturbance—role failure, role loss, interpersonal role conflict, or role insufficiency—*to assess limitations and plan strategies to cope with role changes.*
Discusses role expectations and changed role performance with significant others	
Uses constructive strategies to cope with situational transition	Determine role of patient within family and social network *to identify expectations.*
Expresses satisfaction with newly acquired functional role performance	Determine scope and nature of situational transition experienced *to assess degree of crisis created by changes.*
Seeks assistance from appropriate resources	Determine cultural factors influencing role expectations and performance.
	Determine patient's expectations of role performance and perceived rewards from role behaviors and clarify any misconceptions about changed functioning *to reinforce reality and decrease denial.*
	Encourage patient to express concerns and feelings about loss of physical health.
	Assist patient in identifying and implementing strategies to deal with situational transition.
	Teach patient about strategies to cope with physical disability.

*For the patient with chronic obstructive pulmonary disease. *continued.*

Role Performance, Altered—cont'd

ROLE PERFORMANCE, ALTERED

PATIENT GOALS/ EXPECTED OUTCOMES	NURSING INTERVENTIONS/ *SCIENTIFIC RATIONALE*
	Assist patient in identifying strengths and resources, including positive role models, *to increase social support and reinforce functional role performance.*
	Discuss impact of role change with family and significant others *to understand and support role functioning of the patient.*
	Use role playing *to teach new behaviors, provide opportunities for role rehearsal, and reinforce change.*
	Offer praise and support for initiating and practicing new behaviors *to build positive self-concept.*

References 21, 26, 73, 225, 278, 287a, 288, 431, 496, 526, 629.

Self-Care Deficit (Bathing/Hygiene, Dressing/Grooming, Feeding, Toileting)

Related factors: Intolerance to activity; decreased strength and endurance

Jin Hee Kim, Rosemarie Suhayda, and Mi Ja Kim

PATIENT GOALS/ EXPECTED OUTCOMES	NURSING INTERVENTIONS/ *SCIENTIFIC RATIONALE*
Perform self-care activities with minimal energy expenditure and risk of injury as evidenced by the following:	
Completes self-care activities without significant changes in baseline vital signs or threat to safety	Assist patient with self-care activities as necessary. Determine energy requirements of self-care activity; identify sources of excessive energy expenditure (length of time and effort required to complete activity; muscle groups involved; ambient environmental conditions). Monitor activity tolerance; *heart rate may be a more sensitive indicator of poorly spaced rest periods than other physiological measures.* Keep needed objects within easy reach.
Carries out bathing and proper toilet hygiene; washes body or body parts	Assist patient with positioning for bathing, eating, grooming, and so on, to avoid awkward postures. Assist with those activities patient is unable to perform himself/herself, such as brushing teeth, combing and shampooing hair, cleaning nails, and bathing back/legs/feet.
Puts on or takes off necessary items of clothing	Provide slightly larger than regular size clothing with modified fasteners, such as velcro closings, zippers, elastic waist, or large neck.

continued.

Self-Care Deficit (Bathing/Hygiene, Dressing/ Grooming, Feeding, Toileting)—cont'd

PATIENT GOALS/ EXPECTED OUTCOMES	NURSING INTERVENTIONS/ *SCIENTIFIC RATIONALE*
	Encourage patient to dress self with assistance of retrieving clothing from closet and/or lay out clothing in appropriate order.
	Allow time to perform each task of dressing and grooming; avoid rushing patient.
Brings food from receptacle to mouth	Provide types of food best handled by patient: finger foods, soft or liquid diet.
	Assist patient with set-up at each meal, such as cutting food into small pieces, opening containers and napkins, buttering bread, pouring drinks, and opening condiment packages.
	Assist patient in his/her normal eating position suited to his/ her physical ability: sitting in a chair at table or high Fowler's position in bed.
	Provide adaptive eating utensils, such as hand splints.
	Provide adequate amount of space in performing the eating task by appropriate food arrangement on table.
Sits on or rises from toilet or commode Manages clothing for toileting	Provide specialized assistive devices, such as tub transfer seat, grab bars, or raised toilet seat, *to enhance ability to move/perform activities safely.*
	Provide bedside commode, bedpan, or urinal.

Self-Care Deficit (Bathing/Hygiene, Dressing/ Grooming, Feeding, Toileting)—cont'd

PATIENT GOALS/ EXPECTED OUTCOMES	NURSING INTERVENTIONS/ *SCIENTIFIC RATIONALE*
	Monitor and take precautions to protect from safety hazards; clear pathways to toilet area; keep bathroom lights on at night; ensure easy access to bathroom.
	With patient, develop individualized activity schedule to achieve goals and monitor progress with frequent feedback to increase compliance.
	Include significant others when appropriate.
	Schedule frequent, short pauses or rest periods.
	Rearrange schedule to reduce energy loss.
	Within tolerance levels and unless contraindicated, begin graduated exercise program. *Exercise may lessen feelings of fatigue.*
	Provide activities designed to stimulate patient's thought process and involvement.
	Encourage maximal independence.
	Teach and encourage patient to participate in self-care activities.
	Monitor underlying cause(s) of activity intolerance, such as prolonged alteration in nutrition, rest/sleep, or work/activity pattern; pain; depression; drug response; pathological condition.

continued.

Self-Care Deficit (Bathing/Hygiene, Dressing/ Grooming, Feeding, Toileting)—cont'd

PATIENT GOALS/ EXPECTED OUTCOMES	NURSING INTERVENTIONS/ *SCIENTIFIC RATIONALE*
	Anticipate activity intolerance in high-risk patient, such as patient's experiencing situational and developmental stressors. Maintain adequate intake of nutrients. Provide frequent, small meals/snacks. Provide aesthetic ambience.

References 98, 150, 161, 270, 547.

Self-Esteem Disturbance

Related factors: Disabling illness; reduced self-care ability*
Gertrude K. McFarland and Elizabeth Kelchner Gerety

PATIENT GOALS/ EXPECTED OUTCOMES	NURSING INTERVENTIONS/ SCIENTIFIC RATIONALE
Experience and maintain self-esteem as evidenced by the following: Differentiates between relationships that reinforce positive feelings vs. relationships that decrease feelings of worth Engages in activities and groups that promote feelings of belonging and acceptance Achieves goals within family and social environment that reflect awareness of personal talents and limitations.	Convey respect and nonjudgmental acceptance of patient as a person. *Creating an atmosphere of acceptance and interest is important so that the patient can begin to explore presenting problems and the significance of current experiences.* Acknowledge patient's expertise or knowledge. Help patient to describe effects of illness on self-appraisal, daily activities, family, and friends. *Illnesses accompanied by functional incapacities may be associated with low levels of self-esteem.* Allow patient to talk about illness *to encourage acceptance of reality of illness. Patients who accept the reality of the disease and integrate this reality into their own self-concept experience higher levels of self-esteem.* Monitor extent to which patient's family influences patient's perception of self. Encourage patient to identify existing strengths and potentials *in order to use these strengths and to reinforce self-esteem.*

*For the elderly patient recently diagnosed with rheumatoid arthritis.

continued.

Self-Esteem Disturbance—cont'd

SELF-ESTEEM DISTURBANCE

PATIENT GOALS/ EXPECTED OUTCOMES	NURSING INTERVENTIONS/ SCIENTIFIC RATIONALE
	Discourage ruminations on past problems and failures.
	Teach family members to recognize the influence of their interactive style on patient's perceptions of self.
	Encourage decision making in planning and directing own care. *Strengthening a coping response and decreasing the patient's tendency to avoid problems or stressors can enhance patient's self-esteem.*
	Encourage patient to initiate activities in which success can be anticipated, *because failure and negative feedback from others can influence one's own self-confidence.*
	Teach patient to create relationships that provide successful social interaction.
	Encourage participation in treatment modalities that emphasize support, acceptance, and belonging.
	Help patient set initial goals that can be achieved within a short period.
	Inspire hope by describing situations in which other patients have managed similar difficulties.

Self-Esteem Disturbance—cont'd

PATIENT GOALS/ EXPECTED OUTCOMES	NURSING INTERVENTIONS/ *SCIENTIFIC RATIONALE*
	Help patient strengthen coping skills and become involved in actions to meet goals within the patient's functional capacity. *Strengthening a coping response, thereby lessening the patient's disposition to avoid problems or stressors, can enhance self-esteem.* Teach meditation/relaxation skills *to provide the patient with the ability to cope with stressors and improve his/her self-esteem and life satisfactions.*
Develop self-care skills necessary for functioning in society as evidenced by the following: Identifies symptoms and accurately reporting them Responds appropriately to emergency situations Maintains good grooming and personal hygiene practices	Monitor ongoing pain levels and follow prescribed guidelines for pain management. Encourage patient to participate in a treatment modality, such as an ADL group or outpatient rehabilitation program, that focuses on learning or relearning how to live independently in a community and achieving highest level of functional capacity. *Maintaining optimal level of health and functioning aids in maintaining patient's self-esteem, as well as optimal social functioning.*
Engages in daily activities to meet personal needs (e.g., meal preparation, home maintenance, planning leisure time)	Emphasize health and personal hygiene, housing, meal planning and preparation, money management, and leisure time.

References 24, 43, 124, 371, 429, 430, 496, 575, 607.

Self-Esteem, Chronic Low

Related factors: Repeated negative and stressful interpersonal relationships

Joan M. Caley and Gertrude K. McFarland

PATIENT GOALS/ EXPECTED OUTCOMES	NURSING INTERVENTIONS/ *SCIENTIFIC RATIONALE*
Develop more positive self-evaluations as evidenced by the following: Decreases number of self-negating statements Evaluates self as able to deal with events Participates in plans to assess, change, and improve self-evaluation	Explore with patient nature of feelings about self and extent of their existence and change over time *to understand the associations of repeated negative interpersonal statements and current state of low self-esteem.* Help patient describe experiences that make him/her feel worthwhile and good about himself/herself. Demonstrate empathy. Provide accurate feedback and give honest answers to questions. Be genuinely interested in and concerned about patient. Be nonjudgmental. *These actions create a supportive reality-based environment for effective problem solving and feedback.*
Engage in constructive interpersonal relationships as evidenced by the following: Demonstrates assertive behavior Engages in meaningful conversation Develops positive interpersonal relationships Evaluates self as able to deal with interpersonal relationships	Observe pattern of interactions with others. Help patient to identify problems in relating to others. Suggest that patient keep journal to assist in problem solving and obtaining feedback.

Self-Esteem, Chronic Low—cont'd

PATIENT GOALS/ EXPECTED OUTCOMES	NURSING INTERVENTIONS/ *SCIENTIFIC RATIONALE*
	Teach patient strategies to improve interpersonal relationships, such as building self-confidence, developing communication skills, making constructive use of defenses, developing hobbies and interests, and developing personal opinions about issues, along with ability to express self assertively to others.
	Assist patient in setting realistic goals to improve interpersonal relationships.
	Role play a variety of ordinary interpersonal encounters.
	Discourage rumination about past failures.
	Encourage participation in recommended support groups.
	These actions promote self-awareness to enhance self-evaluation and encourage self-care. In addition, they help the patient learn new skills in establishing and maintaining constructive interpersonal relationships.

continued.

PATIENT GOALS/ EXPECTED OUTCOMES	NURSING INTERVENTIONS/ *SCIENTIFIC RATIONALE*
Develop more healthful physical life-style as evidenced by the following: Suffers no accidents or injuries Decreases risk for illness Increases ability to understand relationship between physical health and positive self-evaluation Participates in planning to make life-style changes to enhance physical health and well-being	Assess patient's current physical health status. Teach patient about relationship between physical health and positive feelings about self. Assist patient in identifying ways to promote health and well-being. Reinforce health-promoting practices, such as exercise, relaxation, and diversional activity. *These actions promote awareness of positive relationship between self-esteem and physical health.*

References 25, 56, 80, 123, 131, 142, 209, 465, 554, 578.

Self-Esteem, Situational Low

Related factors: Organizational instability; impending job loss
Gertrude K. McFarland and Joan M. Caley

PATIENT GOALS/ EXPECTED OUTCOMES	NURSING INTERVENTIONS/ *SCIENTIFIC RATIONALE*
Regain previous positive self-esteem as evidenced by the following:	
Decreases negative feelings about self	Help patient to identify changes in feelings about self.
Increases confidence in handling job situation	Assist patient in clearly describing previous state of positive self-evaluation.
Increases use of constructive conflict-resolution skills	Explore with patient current employment organizational environment (e.g., degree of organizational instability, level of interpersonal conflict, impending threat to current job).
Increases ability to problem solve, set goals, and take action	Help patient to assess realistic options for self within current organization and other potential employment opportunities, short-term and long-term.
Increases understanding of situational factors and self-behaviors that have an impact on current situation	Engage patient in problem solving (e.g., assess realities of situation, examine personal assets and strengths, identify incremental goals, develop action plan to meet goals).
	These actions promote awareness of positive relationship between self-esteem and effective problem solving.
	Review with patient community groups that could help patient with problem solving and decision making about transitions.
	Offer patient reading materials that might assist in problem solving.
	Teach patient awareness of potential harmful effects of negative self-talk.

continued.

Self-Esteem, Situational Low—cont'd

PATIENT GOALS/ EXPECTED OUTCOMES	NURSING INTERVENTIONS/ *SCIENTIFIC RATIONALE*
	Teach conflict-resolution skills. Teach patient defenses against attacks from others. Refer to resources available in identifying job opportunities. *These actions encourage self-care skills to enhance self-esteem.* Assist patient in describing current level of on-the-job performance and any impact on other aspects of daily living. Help patient to identify previous problem-solving strategies and strengths, limitations, and potentials. Offer hope that situation can be handled by describing others who have overcome similar job instabilities. Suggest that patient keep journal to assist in problem solving and obtaining feedback. Support patient's decision-making efforts. *These actions create a supportive reality-based environment for effective problem solving and feedback.*
Maintain physical health as evidenced by the following: Experiences no accidents or injuries Decreases risk for illness Improves balance between physical and mental health states Participates in planning to make life-style changes to enhance physical health and well-being	Assess patient's current physical health status. Teach patient about relationship between physical health and positive feelings about self. Assist patient in identifying ways to promote health and well-being.

Self-Esteem, Situational Low—cont'd

PATIENT GOALS/ EXPECTED OUTCOMES	NURSING INTERVENTIONS/ SCIENTIFIC RATIONALE
	Reinforce health-promoting practices, such as exercise, relaxation, and diversional activity. *These actions promote awareness of positive relationship between self-esteem and physical health.*

References 24, 25, 56, 80, 123, 131, 142, 199, 325, 578, 602.

SELF-MUTILATION, HIGH RISK FOR

Risk factor: Borderline personality
Gertrude K. McFarland and Charlotte E. Naschinski

PATIENT GOALS/ EXPECTED OUTCOMES	NURSING INTERVENTIONS/ *SCIENTIFIC RATIONALE*
Experience fewer episodes of self-mutilation as evidenced by the following:	
Identifies and manages anxiety	Develop trusting relationship with patient.
Constructively uses resources to deal with stressors	Create non-threatening environment, *because an increase in stressors can lead to self-mutilation.*
Demonstrates self-differentiation	
Makes positive self-statements	
Displays positive family interactions	Assist patient in recognition of anxiety and situations in which he/she becomes anxious. This essential step is necessary before plans for reducing anxiety can be developed.
	Explore with patient approaches to reduce anxiety (e.g., music, physical activity).
	Assist patient to identify perceived stressors.
	Explore with patient past successes in reducing stress *to capitalize use of patient's strengths.*
	Collaborate with patient to develop a plan to cope with stressors.
	Have patient demonstrate use of stress-reduction techniques.
	Engage patient in values clarification, self-appraisal, and identification of ideal self *to develop clearer sense of self-identity.*

Self-Mutilation, High Risk for—cont'd

PATIENT GOALS/ EXPECTED OUTCOMES	NURSING INTERVENTIONS/ SCIENTIFIC RATIONALE
	Provide opportunities in which patient can maximize use of his/her strengths *to enhance self-esteem.*
	Offer unconditional positive regard when interacting with patient *to enhance feelings of self-esteem.*
	Determine to what extent the patient's self-perception is affected by his/her dysfunctional family.
	Discuss alternative strategies with patient to enhance family interaction (e.g., family therapy) *so as to decrease any stress or threat to self.*

References 118, 168, 169, 173, 608.

Sensory/Perceptual Alterations (Auditory)

Related factors: Traumatic emotional events*
Evelyn L. Wasli and Gertrude K. McFarland

PATIENT GOALS/ EXPECTED OUTCOMES	NURSING INTERVENTIONS/ *SCIENTIFIC RATIONALE*

Experience reduction in hallucinations as evidenced by the following:
Recognizes that hallucinations are a part of patient's experience and can be dealt with
Develops psychosocial strategies to relieve the stress or manage the behaviors and/or feelings resulting from the experiences of hallucinations
	Develop supportive environment and therapeutic nurse-patient relationship *to enhance comfort level and reduce anxiety in patient.*
	    Be available for patient in a variety of daily living situations so that he/she can explore experiences.
	    Avoid suggesting that a voice is actually being heard.
	    Assist in identifying what, who, when, where, and how of the auditory hallucinations.
	Assist patient in developing a frame of reference for understanding the voices *to promote coping and to reduce hallucinations.*
	Provide information to patient about nature of hallucinations, their relationship to stressor/traumatic emotional events, treatments, and ways of coping *to assist patient in understanding hallucinations.*
	Teach patient strategies to decrease stress *to reduce need for hallucinations.*
	Teach patient strategies to deal with other social contexts in which hallucinations are experienced.

*For the patient with schizophrenia experiencing auditory hallucinations.

Sensory/Perceptual Alterations (Auditory)—cont'd

PATIENT GOALS/ EXPECTED OUTCOMES	NURSING INTERVENTIONS/ *SCIENTIFIC RATIONALE*
	Teach use of diversional activities (e.g., tapes, enjoyable events). Provide patient opportunity to exchange experiences with others.

References 280, 282, 373, 422, 501.

Sexual Dysfunction

Related factors: Misinformation or inadequate knowledge; conflicting values
Gertrude K. McFarland and Karen V. Scipio-Skinner

PATIENT GOALS/ EXPECTED OUTCOMES	NURSING INTERVENTIONS/ SCIENTIFIC RATIONALE
Verbalize increased knowledge about sexual concerns as evidenced by the following:	
Identifies personal sexual concerns	Encourage patient to describe current sexual interactions and behavior patterns (e.g., compatibility with sexual partner; comfort with sexual interactions; frequency of sexual interactions). *Patients need reassurance from authoritative source that it is permissible to think, read, talk, and fantasize about sex.*
	Provide privacy when discussing sexual matters. Provide climate in which patient can openly discuss concerns. Use nonjudgmental attitude. *Comfort factors show respect to client and promote expression of feeling.*
	Acknowledge patient's feelings of anxiety about discussing sexual concerns *to establish rapport and create an internal state of trust for patient.*
Verbalizes knowledge about human sexuality	
	Explore patient's knowledge deficit about sexuality (e.g., How did patient learn about sexuality? What is patient's understanding about normal sexual functions?)

Sexual Dysfunction—cont'd

PATIENT GOALS/ EXPECTED OUTCOMES	NURSING INTERVENTIONS/ *SCIENTIFIC RATIONALE*
	Dispel any myths or misinformation patient may have about sexual activities (e.g., that masturbating will make you crazy). *Patients need to have myths dispelled and be provided with accurate information about sexual functioning.*
	Use terminology that patient understands (e.g., does patient know what the words *coitus* and *sexual intercourse* mean?)
	Clarify with patient any uncertainties about terminology being used (slang or street terminology can have a variety of meanings).
	Because the same words may have different meaning for different people, the nurse must be constantly prepared to define the meaning of a word or phrase.
Identify and discuss personal sexual beliefs and values as evidenced by the following:	
Selects socially acceptable behaviors consistent with personal beliefs and values	Explore with patient beliefs and values regarding sexuality (e.g., How do factors, such as patient's early childhood beliefs, religious beliefs, and perceptions of parental attitudes toward sex affect present beliefs and values?)

continued.

Sexual Dysfunction—cont'd

PATIENT GOALS/ EXPECTED OUTCOMES	NURSING INTERVENTIONS/ *SCIENTIFIC RATIONALE*
	Within own scope of knowledge and level of comfort, offer suggestions to patient about alternative sexual behaviors or outlets. Allow patient the opportunity to discuss suggestions. *Make facts available whenever patient needs or asks for them; this builds trust, orients, enables decision making, and decreases anxiety, frustration, or other distressing feelings that hinder realistic action, thereby helping the patient focus on deeper concerns.*
	Provide specific facts that address expressed needs.
	Listen to what the patient has to say without jumping to conclusions or interpreting behavior prematurely. *Careful listening conveys respect and promotes self-esteem and a sense of security and safety.*
	Attend closely to verbal and nonverbal signals suggesting anxiety or indications that a problem is more extensive than originally presented. Encourage communications between partners. Recommend a self-help program or refer to individual or group counseling, as appropriate. *Nonverbal behavior often conveys more directly the feelings and is often the key to the message.*

Sexual Dysfunction—cont'd

PATIENT GOALS/ EXPECTED OUTCOMES	NURSING INTERVENTIONS/ *SCIENTIFIC RATIONALE*
	Assist the patient in describing behavior rather than labeling (e.g., "I have difficulty becoming sexually aroused" instead of "I am frigid"). Help the patient determine whether a behavior is helpful or useful in reaching goals, instead of labeling behavior as good or bad. *Patients need help in arriving at their own answers and determining what is right or wrong; do not judge for the patient what is right or wrong, normal or abnormal. Patients must decide what is normal for them.*
	Teach patient assertive communication skills so that patient can say "no" or not do something. *Assertiveness training provides the patient with the behavioral repertoire needed to successfully interact with others.*

References 22, 84, 204, 250, 275, 333, 413.

Related factors: Knowledge/skill deficit about medical treatment*

Carol Kupperberg and Gertrude K. McFarland

PATIENT GOALS/ EXPECTED OUTCOMES	NURSING INTERVENTIONS/ *SCIENTIFIC RATIONALE*
Attain satisfying level of sexual activity compatible with functional capacity as evidenced by the following: Resumes sexual activity at or near premorbid level at time determined by individual limiting factors	Provide specific information to patient and partner about limitations; correct myths and misinformation; address issues with sensitivity to customs and cultural issues. *Patients who receive education and counseling report improved sexual satisfaction and performance due to decreased anxiety.* Use information about premorbid sexual activity obtained through sexual history as basis for teaching and counseling; assess for long-standing sexual dysfunction, which can be caused by a psychogenic problem rather than physical illness, medication, or organic problem. *Assessment of patterns of sexual activity provides basis for individualized counseling and can help identify previous patterns that caused physiological and psychological stress.*

*For the patient with myocardial infarction.

PATIENT GOALS/ EXPECTED OUTCOMES	NURSING INTERVENTIONS/ *SCIENTIFIC RATIONALE*
	Examine concerns about sexuality and adequacy of sexual function. *Issues that may influence resumption of sexual activity are fear of sudden death or precipitation of symptoms such as angina, dyspnea, and palpitations; perceived change in body image; depression, which can affect ability to invest emotionally and be a factor in sexual dysfunction; forced dependency; changes in feelings of self-worth; and attractiveness to sexual partner.*
	Assess level of comfort in discussing topic alone or with partner; provide opportunity for both. *Individual counseling allows discussion of issues that may cause discomfort if discussed with partner present (e.g., concerns about extramarital sexual relationships or concerns about coital death).*
	Address stress, fears, and sexual concerns of partner and examine relationship with sexual partner. *Partner should be included in the counseling process; if not he/she may become overprotective and seek to limit those activities that are seen as potentially harmful to patient.*

continued.

Sexuality Patterns, Altered—cont'd

SEXUALITY PATTERNS, ALTERED

PATIENT GOALS/ EXPECTED OUTCOMES	NURSING INTERVENTIONS/ *SCIENTIFIC RATIONALE*
	Teach patient about possible side effects of drugs such as digitalis, hypnotics, tranquilizers, and diuretics. *Commonly prescribed medications may affect libido and cause inorgasmia and/or erectile problems.*
	Assess physical status, that indicates when sexual activity can be safely resumed: patient's general health, tolerance for physical activity before MI, extent of myocardial damage, frequency and severity of angina or arrythmias, and patient's ability to tolerate progression of activity. *Base advice to patient on consultation with physician. Depending on individual case, patient may resume sexual intercourse 3 to 6 weeks after MI.*
	Before discharge, evaluate physical status with low-level treadmill test, portable ECG recording made during moderate exercise, or by two-flight stair-climbing test followed by resting ECG recording. *The peripheral O_2 demands of intercourse are in the 4 to 5 MET (metabolic equivalent) range. The ability to exercise at 5 or 6 METs and attain a heart rate of 115 to 120 beats/minute without such symptoms as ischemic changes or significant arrythmias signifies that resumption of sexual activity will be safe.*

PATIENT GOALS/ EXPECTED OUTCOMES	NURSING INTERVENTIONS/ *SCIENTIFIC RATIONALE*
	Assist patient in developing individualized plan of progressive physical and sexual activity based on physiological limitations. *Sexual activity should be resumed gradually. Similar to any physical activity, sexual intercourse places increased demands on the cardiovascular system.*
	Instruct about potential for angina during sexual intercourse and how to respond (stop; take nitroglycerine; may resume after relief is obtained). *If couple is advised that angina may occur and they know what to do, they may be better able to cope if they do encounter this problem. Additional medication may be needed to prevent angina.*
	Advise patient to avoid sexual activity for 2 or more hours after eating. *Angina may occur due to increased blood flow to GI organs and increased demands caused by sexual activity. This results in decreased blood flow to myocardium.*
	Advise patient to avoid sexual activity after excessive alcohol intake. *Alcohol causes decreased cardiac output, which may decrease the amount of exercise that can be performed without provoking angina.*

continued.

SEXUALITY PATTERNS, ALTERED

PATIENT GOALS/ EXPECTED OUTCOMES	NURSING INTERVENTIONS/ *SCIENTIFIC RATIONALE*
	Teach patient warning signs that must be reported to physician: rapid pulse or respiratory rate that persists 4 to 5 minutes after orgasm, feeling of extreme fatigue after sexual activity, anginal symptoms during or after sexual activity. *Potentially significant dysrhythmias and arrhythmias can be precipitated by sexual activity. Cardiovascular symptoms that occur during sexual activity may require further evaluation, use of medication, and physical conditioning, which would allow the patient to exercise in greater comfort.*

References 34, 90, 203, 310, 360, 399, 514, 570.

Skin Integrity, Impaired

Related factors: Physical immobilization; altered circulation*
Kathryn Czurylo and Mi Ja Kim

PATIENT GOALS/ EXPECTED OUTCOMES	NURSING INTERVENTIONS/ SCIENTIFIC RATIONALE
Have intact skin in area of disruption as evidenced by the following:	
Skin lesion is clean and healing	Perform assessment of wound (stage 1-4) and surrounding skin as a baseline and document regularly.
Patient/significant other demonstrates proper skin care	Keep skin clean and dry.
Decreased pressure to integument	Perform prescribed dressing changes at site of lesion.
Circulation to integument is maintained	Debride and clean wound as ordered.
Lab values are within normal limits	Provide wound treatment (e.g., per order—ointments, plastic coatings, gauze, nonabsorptive thin films, absorptive thick wafers, absorptive gels, enzymatic debriding agents, lubricating spray).
	Monitor patient closely for signs and symptoms of infection: fever, drainage, pain, anorexia.
	Instruct patient/significant other about the following and have him/her return demonstrate: Skin inspection Wound care as ordered Keeping skin clean Skin lubrication Protection from environmental agents Skin massage and position changes

*For the patient with pressure ulcer.

continued.

SKIN INTEGRITY, IMPAIRED

PATIENT GOALS/ EXPECTED OUTCOMES	NURSING INTERVENTIONS/ SCIENTIFIC RATIONALE
	When to contact physician: signs and symptoms of infection, worsening wound condition, new lesion
	Keeping pressure off lesion
	Ambulate patient if possible.
	When patient is in bed, turn every 1 to 2 hours; use all four sides if possible (lateral, prone, dorsal), avoiding positioning on lesion.
	Teach patient to change position if possible.
	Use low-air-loss therapy or air-fluidized therapy bed.
	Massage skeletal prominences with lotion every 2 hours.
	Do not massage reddened areas *because rubbing may cause additional trauma.*
	Prevent head of bed (HOB) elevation of more than 30 degrees for long periods. *Shearing forces are generated on sacrum, causing mechanical stress.*
	Avoid use of doughnuts and rubber rings *because these increase pressure and damage tissue.*
	Provide the following:
	Increased calories and protein. *Tissues are more vulnerable to necrosis with smaller amounts of pressure if the diet is deficient in these.*
	Fluid intake adequate to prevent dehydration (2600 ml/ day if possible).

Skin Integrity, Impaired—cont'd

PATIENT GOALS/ EXPECTED OUTCOMES	NURSING INTERVENTIONS/ *SCIENTIFIC RATIONALE*
	Iron and vitamin C supplements as needed. *Vitamin C is important for wound healing, fosters collagen synthesis and capillary function; iron improves oxygen-carrying capacity of blood.*
	Monitor lab values that have an impact on skin and report abnormalities:
	Hct/Hgb; *low levels compromise oxygen delivery to tissues.*
	BUN; *elevated levels may indicate renal disease, which may affect albumin.*
	Albumin; *low amounts cause interstitial edema, which impedes exchange to nutrients and waste products.*
	Bilirubin; *elevated levels may indicate liver disease, which may affect albumin.*
	Arterial blood gases (ABGs); *indicates oxygen available for tissues.*
	Perform passive ROM every 2 hours, *which promotes circulation to area of lesion.*

References 38, 54, 122, 136, 182, 210, 252, 341, 347, 414, 634.

Risk factor: Prolonged bedrest*
Kathryn Czurylo and Mi Ja Kim

PATIENT GOALS/ EXPECTED OUTCOMES	NURSING INTERVENTIONS/ SCIENTIFIC RATIONALE
Maintain intact skin tissue as evidenced by the following:	
Experiences no broken skin	Keep skin clean and dry after washing.
Experience less pressure to integument as evidenced by the following:	Prevent extremes in environmental temperature and humidity.
No reddened areas	Monitor patient for the following risk factors:
Maintain adequate circulation to integument as evidenced by the following:	Incontinence
	Immobility
No reddened areas	Inactivity
No cyanosis	Poor nutrition
Patient/significant other returns demonstration of proper skin care	Poor hydration
	Edema
	Monitor blood chemistry levels that have an impact on skin, and report abnormalities when present:
	Hct/Hbg; *low levels compromise oxygen delivery to the tissue.*
	BUN; *elevated levels may indicate renal disease, which may affect albumin.*
	Albumin; *low amounts cause interstitial edema, which impedes exchange of nutrients and waste products.*
	Bilirubin; *elevated levels may indicate liver disease, which may affect albumin.*
	Arterial blood gases (ABGs); *indicates oxygen available for tissues.*

*For the patient with an acute CVA.

Skin Integrity, Impaired, High Risk for—cont'd

PATIENT GOALS/ EXPECTED OUTCOMES	NURSING INTERVENTIONS/ *SCIENTIFIC RATIONALE*
	Instruct patient/significant other about the following and have him/her return demonstration: Skin inspection for redness, cyanosis, blistering, temperature, and pulses Keeping skin clean Skin lubrication Protection from environmental agents Skin massage and position changes When to contact physician: skin reddening, breakdown Keeping pressure off skin and skeletal prominences as much as possible Ambulate patient if possible. When patient is in bed, turn every 1-2 hours; use all four sides (lateral, prone, dorsal), unless contraindicated. Teach patient to change position, if possible. Use static devices (foam or water, air, or gel-filled) as necessary. Massage skeletal prominences with lotion every 2 hours. Do not massage reddened areas *because rubbing may cause additional trauma.* Prevent head of bed (HOB) elevation of more than 30 degrees for long periods. *Shearing forces are generated on sacrum, causing mechanical stress.*

continued.

SKIN INTEGRITY, IMPAIRED, HIGH RISK FOR

PATIENT GOALS/ EXPECTED OUTCOMES	NURSING INTERVENTIONS/ *SCIENTIFIC RATIONALE*
	Avoid use of doughnuts and rubber rings *because these increase pressure and damage tissue.*
	Provide adequate nutrition, including the following:
	Sufficient calories and protein. *Tissues are more vulnerable to necrosis with smaller amounts of pressure if the diet is deficient in calories and protein.*
	Fluid intake adequate to prevent dehydration (2600 ml/day if possible).
	Have patient do active ROM, or do passive ROM for patient, every 2 hours *to promote circulation to skin and to alter weight-bearing.*
	Elevate legs to prevent edema. *Edema slows oxygen diffusion and metabolic transport from capillary to cell.*

References 49, 104, 117, 136, 348, 637.

Sleep Pattern Disturbance

Related factors: Disruptions in life-style or usual sleep habits during illness or hospitalization
Susan Dudas and Mi Ja Kim

PATIENT GOALS/ EXPECTED OUTCOMES	NURSING INTERVENTIONS/ SCIENTIFIC RATIONALE
Understand factors contributing to sleep pattern disturbances as evidenced by the following:	
Participates in determining potential causes for inadequate sleep	Compare patient's current sleep pattern with usual sleep habits before hospitalization or current episode of sleep disturbance.
	Monitor and discuss possible causes for disturbed sleep (e.g., patient's worries, concerns, pain).
	Encourage expression of concerns if and when patient is unable to sleep.
	Confer with family/significant others about potential causes of sleep pattern disturbance.
	Evaluate effects of patient's medications (e.g., steroids, diuretics) that may interfere with sleep. *Psychic derangements may occur when corticosteroids are used, including mood swings, insomnia, and so on.*
	Observe and monitor patient's daytime habits/activities.
Verbalizes understanding of specific plan to manage or correct causes of inadequate sleep	Plan daytime activities.
	Discourage daytime napping *only* if daytime naps negatively affect nighttime sleep. *Unsynchronized circadian sleep-wake cycles result from short naps dispersed over a 24-hour period.*

continued.

Sleep Pattern Disturbance—cont'd

PATIENT GOALS/ EXPECTED OUTCOMES	NURSING INTERVENTIONS/ SCIENTIFIC RATIONALE
	Monitor patient to avoid excessive time in bed (if medically appropriate).
Sleep through the night or at least for increased lengths of uninterrupted periods as evidenced by the following: Falls asleep within 30 to 45 minutes of going to bed	Determine patient's usual nighttime habits and provide for routine as closely as possible (e.g., provide warm milk if allowed on medical regimen and if no nighttime voiding problem exists). *Changing a person's usual pattern of food intake in the evening has been found to impair subsequent sleep.* Decrease fluid intake before bedtime (if wakening for frequent voiding occurs). Have patient empty bladder at bedtime. Avoid caffeine for 4 hours before sleep (if fluids are needed, substitute decaffeinated drinks). Promote relaxation at bedtime: select interventions approved by patient (e.g., provide soft music; provide back massage; suggest guided imagery techniques; teach muscle relaxation techniques).

Sleep Pattern Disturbance—cont'd

PATIENT GOALS/ EXPECTED OUTCOMES	NURSING INTERVENTIONS/ SCIENTIFIC RATIONALE
	Provide patient with comfortable environment to promote sleep or rest (e.g., turn off lights; provide adequate room ventilation; provide warmth or coolness as needed; avoid noise disturbances). *Cortical inhibition on reticular formation is eliminated during sleep, enhancing autonomic responses; thus cardiovascular responses to noise are greater during sleep.*
	Avoid strenuous physical or mental activity just before bedtime.
	Schedule assessments or interventions to allow for longer sleep periods (e.g., check vital signs and turn patient at same time). *Sleep deprivation occurs with frequent interruption of sleep and may impair recovery due to psychological and physiological disturbances. Patient's own circadian rhythm is disturbed by interruptions.*
Minimal number of essential interruptions occur	Help patient to maintain a normal day/night pattern to facilitate night sleeping.
Sleeps during longer intervals between nursing care functions	Provide sedation as prescribed, if necessary, temporarily.
Verbalizes feeling of being rested or refreshed	Determine effectiveness of sedative prescribed (i.e., optimal dosage, no rebound effects).
	Monitor level of daytime alertness.

References 4, 42, 148, 211, 237, 331, 405, 493, 580, 586, 627.

Related factors: Knowledge/skill deficit about ways to enhance mutuality; absence of available significant others

Mary E. Markert and Gertrude K. McFarland

PATIENT GOALS/ EXPECTED OUTCOMES	NURSING INTERVENTIONS/ SCIENTIFIC RATIONALE
Increase social competence as evidenced by the following:	
Increases ability to cope with interpersonal encounters and social situations	Assess with patient factors contributing to difficulty in social interactions.
	Observe patient for interaction style.
Expresses feelings in a socially acceptable manner	Review patterns of relating with family/peers and coping skills.
	Encourage patient to express feelings and perceptions of social skills.
	These actions provide information about socialization skills, interaction style, and perception of social adequacy.
	Employ brief contacts at frequent intervals.
	Discuss neutral topics or subjects in which patient has an interest.
	Provide opportunities for meaningful task performance within the milieu.
	Provide feedback about observed interactions.
Verbalizes awareness of feelings that lead to poor social relationships	Assist patient with identifying feelings that cause discomfort in social situations.
	Help patient to identify situations in which others are alienated because of patient's behaviors.

Social Interaction, Impaired—cont'd

PATIENT GOALS/ EXPECTED OUTCOMES	NURSING INTERVENTIONS/ *SCIENTIFIC RATIONALE*
	Modeling, structuring, and providing feedback promote awareness of positive actions and problem areas.
Increase interactions with others as evidenced by the following:	
Resumes or adds to socialization activities	Facilitate conversation between patient and peers.
Expresses satisfaction in interpersonal relationships	Help patient to identify others with whom he/she feels comfortable and encourage interactions and activities with them.
	Elicit expressed preference for roommate or activities.
	Structure milieu to promote socialization (small areas for reading, games, refreshments).
	Emphasize attendance at routine activities and resumption of hobbies.
	Encourage visits by friends, relatives.
	These actions reduce isolation and increase potential for successful socialization experiences.
	Use social skills training to assist patient to identify strategies, role play more effective behavior, obtain social reinforcement, and try the behavior in a real situation.
	Help patient move from one-to-one interactions into small-group activities.

continued.

SOCIAL INTERACTION, IMPAIRED

PATIENT GOALS/ EXPECTED OUTCOMES	NURSING INTERVENTIONS/ *SCIENTIFIC RATIONALE*
	Maintain consistent small-group membership so that trust, open sharing, and role identification can occur.
	Use creative activities to provide opportunities for self-expression and demonstration of talent, as well as group interaction.
	Encourage initiative in identifying opportunities for social interaction with friends, family, and community groups.
	These actions provide increased opportunity for feedback and social reinforcement.
	Provide positive reinforcement for demonstration of more effective social skills. *Reinforcement encourages repetition of desired behaviors.*

References 39, 151, 329, 350, 568, 573, 587.

Social Isolation

Related factors: Inability to engage in satisfying personal relationships

Jane Lancour and Audrey M. McLane

PATIENT GOALS/ EXPECTED OUTCOMES	NURSING INTERVENTIONS/ SCIENTIFIC RATIONALE
Develop a trusting relationship as evidenced by the following:	
Demonstrates a trusting relationship by expressing feelings of loneliness, distrust, and sense of self	Facilitate and explore expressions of feelings. Explore dynamics of past relationships: process and outcome. Engage in active listening. Alert patient to negative self-talk and discuss inaccuracies of perception. Complete measurement of loneliness and self-concept inventory. Complete social skills checklist. Provide patient with a summary of key areas in need of improvement. Help patient to recognize bodily reactions to cognitions. *Awareness is a first step in gaining control over thoughts, feelings, and behaviors.*
Reduce degree of social isolation as evidenced by the following:	
Spends one period per week in group therapy Invites one person to visit home within 2-month period Selects and participates in one leisure group activity every 2 weeks	Provide information about available pertinent group therapy (e.g., social skills training, cognitive reappraisal, social support). Develop plan of action with patient.

continued.

SOCIAL ISOLATION

PATIENT GOALS/ EXPECTED OUTCOMES	NURSING INTERVENTIONS/ *SCIENTIFIC RATIONALE*
	Provide positive reinforcement for even the slightest movement away from pattern of social isolation.
	Structure with patient a self-modification program using self-selected strategies.
Develop one or two meaningful relationships as evidenced by the following:	
Identifies two individuals who are important and why they are important	Identify barriers to forming meaningful relationships.
Interacts with these individuals on a regular basis	Discuss relationship of personal responsibility and social isolation.
	Discuss and analyze at each visit positive and negative aspects of interpersonal interactions that occurred in previous week.
	Discuss reality and risks/benefits of opening oneself to others.
Develop interest in volunteering to assist someone or an organization as evidenced by the following:	
Makes one phone call per week for 3 weeks, inquiring about volunteer services	Discuss satisfaction that can be experienced through helping others.
	Provide patient with information about volunteer possibilities in immediate vicinity. *Engaging in volunteer activities provides recognition and allows patient to experience satisfying personal relationships.*

Social Isolation—cont'd

PATIENT GOALS/ EXPECTED OUTCOMES	NURSING INTERVENTIONS/ *SCIENTIFIC RATIONALE*
	Ask patient to make one phone call per week to obtain information about volunteer services and elicit feelings about that phone call at next session.
Expand and engage in new interests as evidenced by the following:	
Engages in one satisfying leisure activity appropriate to developmental stage with another individual(s) on a regular basis	Negotiate with patient to complete a leisure assessment. Explore with patient obstacles to involvement in one leisure activity identified as interesting. Help patient to engage in strategies to overcome obstacles.

References 162, 294, 449, 454, 510, 515, 578.

328

Spiritual Distress (Distress of the Human Spirit)

Related factors: Challenged belief in God; separated from formal religious and family support*
Richard J. Fehring and Audrey M. McLane

PATIENT GOALS/ EXPECTED OUTCOMES	NURSING INTERVENTIONS/ SCIENTIFIC RATIONALE
Improve spiritual well-being as evidenced by the following:	
Achieves high score (80-120) on Spiritual Well-Being Index of Paloutzian and Ellison	Provide models of persons who have overcome difficulties, using examples from literature, Bible, personal experiences, and so on.
Makes positive statements about self and life	Encourage/accept verbalization of feelings of anger.
Articulates and is comfortable with belief system	Teach cognitive strategies (e.g., combating distorted thinking and values clarification). *Clarification of values will help patient develop short-term and long-term goals for spiritual growth.*
	Provide referral to spiritual counselor.
	Monitor spiritual distress with Spiritual Well-Being Index of Paloutzian and Ellison.
	Provide daily prayer/meditation booklet congruent with reading level and expressed religious/denominational preference.
	Use imagery/prayer/music to heal past life hurts.
	Discuss importance of trying new religious exercises more than one time. *Spiritual well-being/distress may differ from day to day; spiritual exercise may not be effective the first time.*

*For a homeless person who believes in God and abuses drugs and alcohol.

Spiritual Distress (Distress of the Human Spirit)—cont'd

PATIENT GOALS/ EXPECTED OUTCOMES	NURSING INTERVENTIONS/ *SCIENTIFIC RATIONALE*
Develop support system with friends/church members as evidenced by the following:	
Initiates ongoing relationship with another individual	Encourage participation in adult prayer, social, and athletic groups.
Feels someone cares about him/her	Use role playing to prepare patient for new relationships.
Participates in group activities (alcohol support group, prayer group, and so on)	
Participate in alcohol rehabilitation program as evidenced by the following:	
Enters and adheres to alcohol rehabilitation program	Refer and advocate patient's entrance into in-patient alcohol and drug treatment program. *Advocacy will help gain entrance into in-patient program, especially if patient has failed in previous out-patient treatment programs.*
Find a job and/or engage in volunteer activity as evidenced by the following:	
Obtains job counseling	Refer to social worker/vocational counselor.
Participates in volunteer program	Explore volunteer opportunities.
Attends basic reading program	Enroll in basic reading program.
Articulates goals in life	*Ongoing social support of case workers and learning basic reading skills will help patient gain self-esteem, establish new goals, and obtain employment.*

References 61, 160, 415, 423, 446, 487, 545, 561, 565.

Risk factors: Periodic emesis after bouts of excessive drinking/ ingestion of a large meal; smokes in bed

Audrey M. McLane

PATIENT GOALS/ EXPECTED OUTCOMES	NURSING INTERVENTIONS/ *SCIENTIFIC RATIONALE*
Recognize increased risk of suffocation as evidenced by the following:	
Permanently removes all smoking materials from bedside	Teach patient dangers of smoking in bed
Establishes a separate area in home for smoking	Use anatomic drawings to teach patient/spouse danger of inhaling expelled gastric contents.
Verbalizes understanding of hazards	
Spouse demonstrates side-lying position and use of supports to keep spouse on side	Teach spouse to position patient on side to avoid inhaling own vomit. *Knowledge of countermeasures will help spouse to reduce risk of suffocation.*
Participate in alcohol rehabilitation program as evidenced by the following:	
Acknowledges drinking problem	Offer patient and spouse opportunity to discuss their perceptions of patient's drinking behavior.
Verbalizes knowledge of adverse effects of drinking	Assist patient in examining consequences of drinking behavior.
Spouse joins Al-Anon Patient enters alcohol treatment program	Provide patient and spouse with list of alcohol treatment programs.

References 166, 175, 519, 577.

Swallowing, Impaired

Related factors: Decreased gag reflex; decreased strength of muscles involved in mastication; decreased oral sensation*
Marilyn Harter, Linda K. Young, Marie Maguire, and
Audrey M. McLane

PATIENT GOALS/ EXPECTED OUTCOMES	NURSING INTERVENTIONS/ *SCIENTIFIC RATIONALE*
Maintain adequate nutritional/hydration status as evidenced by the following:	
Swallows with assistance of verbal cueing	Provide mouth care before and after meals.
Gradually requires fewer verbal cues to swallow	Provide dietary supplements.
Communicates food preferences (may need to use communication board device)	*Oral care and available supplements enhance the likelihood of oral intake.*
	Collaborate with dietitian/ speech therapist to develop plan for introduction and progression of foods and fluids.
	Fluid progression: Introduce thick liquids first. Progressively add thin liquids, beginning with juices with most taste (citrus) and most sensation (carbonated beverages).
	Add thin liquids without much taste last (water, tea, coffee). Always begin with cold liquids and progress to hot. *When swallowing is impaired, swallowing thick liquids is easier than swallowing thin liquids.*

*For the patient who has paralysis of the left side of face and mouth (4 days after CVA). *continued.*

PATIENT GOALS/ EXPECTED OUTCOMES	NURSING INTERVENTIONS/ *SCIENTIFIC RATIONALE*
	Food progression: Introduce foods with pureed consistency first. Progressively add mechanical soft (ground) foods, then solid foods. Begin solid foods with those that require the least chewing. Begin feeding with less than 1 teaspoon of food. *Highly viscous foods increase peristalsis at each meal.* Place foods on unaffected side of mouth. *The client is able to control bolus of food more effectively when it is placed on unaffected side of mouth.* Use verbal cueing (name each bit of food, where placed, and when to swallow). *Cueing provides sequencing for client.* Determine patient's food preferences from patient and family members *to increase the probability of nutritional intake.* Provide high-calorie nutritional supplement 2 hours after meals and at bedtime. *Providing nutritional supplements between meals supports adequate nutritional state.* Monitor intake (calorie estimates, daily weights) and record intake and output. *Monitoring helps determine nutritional and hydration status.*

Swallowing, Impaired—cont'd

PATIENT GOALS/ EXPECTED OUTCOMES	NURSING INTERVENTIONS/ SCIENTIFIC RATIONALE
Improve ability to swallow foods and liquids safely as evidenced by the following: Swallows safely without gagging and without aspirating Nonverbal behaviors suggest increased confidence in swallowing ability	Follow recommendations of speech therapist *to provide consistent approach to facilitate swallowing.* Position patient upright with head flexed slightly forward at mealtimes. Keep in upright position for ½ hour after eating. *This position reduces the possibility of aspiration.* Rotate head toward the affected side. *Rotation causes the bolus to lateralize away from the direction of rotation when swallowing.* Provide rest periods before and during feedings *to ensure maximal participation in eating.* Minimize distractions in the environment *to keep patient focused on sequencing of swallowing.* Teach and reinforce with patient/family that swallowing problems may be temporary. *Accurate information may help the client/family cope with the present impairment.* Praise small gains in ability to swallow. *Positive reinforcement enhances confidence in swallowing.*

continued.

SWALLOWING, IMPAIRED

PATIENT GOALS/ EXPECTED OUTCOMES	NURSING INTERVENTIONS/ SCIENTIFIC RATIONALE
Family members participate in care management as evidenced by the following:	
Family members assist patient with feeding with less supervision over time	Collaborate with speech therapist in teaching swallowing techniques to family members.
Family members describe/demonstrate Heimlich maneuver	Teach Heimlich maneuver to family members *to prepare family for possible emergency situations.*
	Reassure family members about actual/potential improvements in swallowing. *Progress may be slow, so indications reflecting improvement need to be highlighted for family.*
Patient/family members make nutritious dietary selections	Encourage family members to assist patient with selection of nutritious foods.
Family members provide encouragement and support during meals	Establish/maintain private, relaxed atmosphere during meals. *Anxiety and helplessness may contribute to impaired swallowing.*

References 32, 147, 149, 163, 255, 337, 343,459, 544.

Thermoregulation, Ineffective

Related factor: Immature thermoregulatory system*
Kathryn Czurylo and Mi Ja Kim

PATIENT GOALS/ EXPECTED OUTCOMES	NURSING INTERVENTIONS/ SCIENTIFIC RATIONALE
Maintain normothermia as evidenced by the following: No signs or symptoms of hypothermia, such as poor feeding, increased or decreased activity, irritability, lethargy, weak cry, tachypnea, tachycardia, grunting, nasal flaring, or periods of apnea Normothermia Other vital signs within normal limits for patient Serum electrolyte levels and fluid balance within normal limits	Adjust environmental temperature to infant's needs. Adjust infant's temperature, using overhead warmer, warm blankets, and head covering for hypothermia; adjust clothing for hyperthermia. During cooling or rewarming, monitor temperature every 30 minutes. Provide warm oxygen. Administer IV fluids at room temperature. Monitor the following lab values that may be affected by thermal instability: Decreased serum pH level indicates presence of acidosis. *Acidosis may be due to increased oxygen demands to generate heat.* Decreased blood glucose. *Hypoglycemia may be due to increased use of carbohydrate stores in an effort to generate heat.* Monitor for dehydration *due to insensible water loss* and seizures *due to overheating of CNS in hyperthermia and vasodilation during rewarming in hypothermia.* Note and consult physician if signs and symptoms of hypothermia/hyperthermia persist.

*For the patient who is a premature infant.
References 306, 390, 574.

THOUGHT PROCESSES, ALTERED

Related factor: Negative self-evaluation*
Evelyn L. Wasli and Gertrude K. McFarland

PATIENT GOALS/ EXPECTED OUTCOMES	NURSING INTERVENTIONS/ SCIENTIFIC RATIONALE
Achieve positive self-evaluation as evidenced by the following: Demonstrates cognitive ability to track the consequences of certain stressful events (e.g., onset of diabetes) on emotions and thoughts about self Develops strategies to cope with negative self-talk	Develop supportive environment and therapeutic nurse-patient relationship *to reduce anxiety or other emotions, such as anger, and enhance development of a more positive self-evaluation and the ability to reduce psychological conflicts.* Teach patient to monitor self in relation to cause of stress or problem and behaviors occurring as result of inaccurate thoughts, and note changes needed; cause of stress or problem; own behavioral response and feelings (e.g, increased anger and feelings about changes in body from diabetes); and automatic thoughts generated (e.g., "Can't deal with this"). Help patient to determine what is helpful, less helpful, or even harmful. Assist patient in identifying cognitive error used most frequently (e.g., associating events occurring directly to self or occurring because of self; exaggerating or discounting part or all of own experience; making sweeping generalizations; forming inferences without sufficient data; attending to selected aspects of a situation; applying black and white moral judgments).

*For the patient with borderline personality disorder and diabetes.

Thought Processes, Altered—cont'd

PATIENT GOALS/ EXPECTED OUTCOMES	NURSING INTERVENTIONS/ *SCIENTIFIC RATIONALE*
	Help patient learn to watch for own reactions to automatic thoughts.
	Assist patient in exploring appropriateness of goal set for self at present time and for the future.
	Teach patient coping strategies to focus on the behavior (e.g., recording of automatic thoughts; asking another about personal interpretations of situation; relaxation techniques; role playing; and using cognitive process/strategies such as catching and stopping automatic thoughts and active problem solving).
	Teach patient how to make more appropriate self-evaluations by examining consistency of personal thoughts with basic views of life and values and developing own standards.
	Teach patient how to reward self in concrete ways (e.g., going to a special movie), as well as cognitive methods (e.g., "That was a good idea").

References 37, 41, 489, 523, 616, 621, 635, 641.

Tissue Integrity, Impaired

Related factor: Venous pooling
Mary V. Hanley and Mi Ja Kim

PATIENT GOALS/ EXPECTED OUTCOMES	NURSING INTERVENTIONS/ SCIENTIFIC RATIONALE
Attain tissue healing as evidenced by the following:	
Edema surrounding lesion is reduced	Assess lesion for depth (partial or full thickness) and healing phase (e.g., granulation, epithelization).
	Remove constrictive clothing.
	Provide physiological and aseptic environment for lesion.
	Clean lesion with nonirritating solutions.
Wound is free of purulent and necrotic material	Remove purulent drainage and necrotic tissue.
Skin color and temperature are consistent with color and temperature of unaffected extremity	Consult physician concerning debridement strategies.
Skin of lower extremity is intact	Teach patient to perform wound care and to detect symptoms and signs of infection or increased inflammation.
	Teach patient to avoid constrictive clothing (e.g., shoes, stockings, tight-waisted undergarments).
Circulatory exercises and postural maneuvers are performed	Demonstrate and assist patient in performing lower extremity exercises and deep-breathing exercises sequentially and in activating skeletal muscle pump and respiratory pump in lying or standing position.
	Elevate extremity when patient is in sitting position.

Tissue Integrity, Impaired—cont'd

PATIENT GOALS/ EXPECTED OUTCOMES	NURSING INTERVENTIONS/ SCIENTIFIC RATIONALE
	Teach patient to avoid crossing legs. *Gravity affects venous flow and lymph in the lower extremities. Crossing legs impedes venous return and promotes venous stasis, which leads to edema formation and impaired tissue perfusion.*
	Develop an exercise schedule with patient that includes a comfortable combination of walking and rest periods and that avoids standing still for prolonged periods.
	Consult physician about compressive stockings or pneumatic leggings when walking. *If venous insufficiency is severe, chronic ambulatory elastic compression stocking therapy may be used to facilitate venous return, promote healing, and/or prevent recurrence of ulceration.*

References 3, 9, 77, 146, 251, 289, 357, 508, 623, 639.

Tissue Perfusion, Altered (Peripheral)

Related factor: Interruption of arterial flow*
Kathryn Czurylo and Mi Ja Kim

PATIENT GOALS/ EXPECTED OUTCOMES	NURSING INTERVENTIONS/ *SCIENTIFIC RATIONALE*
Manifest decreasing signs and symptoms of tissue damage as evidenced by the following:	
Improvement or maintenance of peripheral circulation as evidenced by decreased claudication, warmth and good color of extremities, and no ulcers Patient/significant other verbalizes knowledge of therapeutic measures Patient/significant other returns demonstration of therapeutic measures, if appropriate	Encourage ambulation, if possible. Instruct on exercise program or active/passive ROM to extremities every 2 hours as appropriate. *Exercise promotes adequate circulation and formation of collateral blood vessels.* Keep legs level with or slightly lower than heart *because gravity promotes arterial circulation and reduces pain.* Avoid prolonged exposure to cold environmental temperature; room temperature should be 72°-74° F. Avoid pressure on extremities by use of heel protectors, water mattress, and foot cradle. Avoid injury to extremities by teaching patient to wear protective shoes and provide good foot care.
Experience less pain as evidenced by the following: Patient verbalizes less pain Decreased use of pain medication	Administer and teach patient about pain medication, vasodilators, and antiplatelet drugs as ordered.

*For the patient with peripheral arterial occlusive disease.

PATIENT GOALS/ EXPECTED OUTCOMES	NURSING INTERVENTIONS/ *SCIENTIFIC RATIONALE*
	Assist patient in controlling risk factors: Smoking; *smoking constricts blood vessels, inhibits ability of blood to carry oxygen by increasing carbon monoxide levels, and results in increased platelet adhesiveness and thrombus formation.* High-fat diet; *lipids attach directly to the arterial wall, causing atherosclerotic lesions.* Sedentary life-style; *sedentary life-style decreases arterial patency and prevents collateral circulation from developing.* Hypertension; *hypertension causes a high-pressure arterial system, which damages the intimal endothelium and makes it more permeable to lipid penetration and plaque formation.* Instruct patient about signs and symptoms to report to physician: cuts, rashes, ulcers, reddened areas, increased pain. Instruct patient/significant other on previously mentioned interventions and have him/her do return demonstration if appropriate. Discuss the patient's/significant others' response to the disease, such as anxiety, powerlessness, depression.

References 40, 53, 58, 154, 170, 242, 396, 591, 608a, 609.

Trauma, High Risk for (Falling)

TRAUMA, HIGH RISK FOR (FALLING)

Risk factors: Cluttered hallways; impaired mobility
Audrey M. McLane

PATIENT GOALS/ EXPECTED OUTCOMES	NURSING INTERVENTIONS/ SCIENTIFIC RATIONALE
Adapt home environment to reduce risk of falling as evidenced by the following:	
Permanently removes all unanchored rugs	Assist patient in examining hazards in environment.
Hallways are clear and well lighted	Identify with patient alternate places to store items in hallways.
	Assist with task of storing items in new locations.
Keeps an updated list of where items are stored	Develop with patient a list of new storage areas.
	Label storage areas and attach list of contents.
Increase activity level as evidenced by the following:	
Obtains and uses walker	Refer patient for free loan of walker from church group.
Walks outdoors when visitors are willing to provide assistance (e.g., open doors)	Teach patient to walk outdoors with visitors (weather permitting).
Increases walking distance 10 ft per week	Develop with patient plan to increase walking distance to tolerance level.
	Demonstrate use of bag on walker to hold portable phone. *Portable phone enables patient to call 911 for help.*

References 243, 267, 274, 279, 426, 477, 577.

Unilateral Neglect

Related factor: Disturbed perceptual ability*
Victoria L. Mock and Gertrude K. McFarland

PATIENT GOALS/ EXPECTED OUTCOMES	NURSING INTERVENTIONS/ SCIENTIFIC RATIONALE
Have realistic awareness of perceptual deficit as evidenced by the following: Verbalizes realistic estimation of degree of deficit—does not ignore or underestimate it	Explain to patient that one side is being neglected Encourage patient to share own perception and provide realistic feedback. *These activities will assist the patient to understand and acknowledge the condition.*
Be protected from injury as evidenced by the following: Experiences no accidents Absence of injury due to deficit	Provide a safe environment by regularly orienting patient to environment; removing excess furniture and equipment; providing good lighting; placing call bell and frequently used objects on unaffected side within easy reach; keeping side rail up on affected side. *Structuring the environment to decrease hazards is essential to safety.* Supervise and/or assist in transferring and ambulating. Protect neglected side during activities and teach patient to assume this responsibility; teach patient to check position of limbs on affected side *to prevent unfelt trauma.*

*For the patient with hemianopia.
continued.

Unilateral Neglect—cont'd

PATIENT GOALS/ EXPECTED OUTCOMES	NURSING INTERVENTIONS/ *SCIENTIFIC RATIONALE*
	Note perceptual deficit on patient record and on patient's room to inform caregivers. *Continuity of safe care is enhanced when all caregivers are aware of the patient's perceptual deficits.*
Acquire knowledge and skill to decrease and/or cope with deficit as evidenced by the following:	
Responds to verbal and/or visual cues to decrease neglect of affected side; scans and protects affected side	Assess regularly for degree of deficit and adaptation to deficit; assess contributing factors.
Compensates for perceptual loss	Initially, assist compensation for perceptual deficit by arranging environment within patient's perceptual field.
Demonstrates increased participation and independence in ADLs	After initial stress, promote conscious attention to neglected side by placing frequently used items on that side; position patient so that affected side is in view; talk to patient from that side.
Verbalizes feeling of progress in regard to perceptual deficit	Spend time with patient, manipulating affected side and encouraging patient to use it.
	Have patient handle ignored limbs with unaffected side.
	Increase stimulation to affected side by touching/massage with scented lotion.
	Use visual and verbal communication regarding limb placement on affected side.

Unilateral Neglect—cont'd

PATIENT GOALS/ EXPECTED OUTCOMES	NURSING INTERVENTIONS/ *SCIENTIFIC RATIONALE*
	Verbal, visual, and tactile cues to decrease neglect of the affected side are effective in enhancing perceptual functioning. Teach patient to scan affected side; place clock or some frequently used item on side of deficit *to help establish a pattern of scanning.* Use "cueing" to affected side (e.g., place red line in margin of books on affected side, small bells on limbs of affected side). Place food tray toward unaffected side; teach patient to rotate plate periodically. Encourage patient to perform ADLs, such as toothbrushing in front of a mirror; supervise and give feedback. *Activities that direct attention to the neglected side can increase awareness and use of that side.* Decrease confusing stimuli; avoid relocation; maintain consistency of caregivers and consistent routine for self-care; explain procedures and treatment well in advance. *An established plan of care by consistent caregivers can decrease distortions in perception and subsequent disorientation.* Include family in rehabilitation process *so that they understand it, support it, and can continue it in home environment.*

References 281, 402, 494, 598, 626, 636.

URINARY ELIMINATION, ALTERED

Related factor: Diminished urinary sphincter control*
Ruth E. McShane and Audrey M. McLane

PATIENT GOALS/ EXPECTED OUTCOMES	NURSING INTERVENTIONS/ SCIENTIFIC RATIONALE
Establish a normal pattern of urinary elimination as evidenced by the following:	
Adheres to established voiding schedule	Teach/monitor use of pelvic floor exercises (PFEs).
Decrease in number of episodes of involuntary loss of urine to occasional loss	Provide written instructions: Sit or stand without tensing muscles of legs, buttocks, or abdomen. Contract and relax circumvaginal muscles and urinary and anal sphincters for 3 to 4 seconds and repeat in a staccato fashion. Do PFEs 25 to 30 times, three times a day. *PFEs strengthen the circumvaginal muscles, urinary sphincter, and external anal sphincter.*
	Establish regular voiding schedule with patient.
Drinks 5 to 6 glasses of water per day	Encourage fluid intake to 1400 ml per day.
	Suggest patient drink 120 ml cranberry juice per day.
Skin in perineal area is clean and dry	Teach patient protective skin care.
No redness or discomfort in perineal area	
Experience decrease in social isolation as evidenced by the following:	
Makes short trips to family member's home	Encourage short visits to friends and relatives.
Reports increase in self-confidence	Suggest regular use of panty liners.
	Encourage patient to contact employer to discuss eventual return to work.

*For the patient with long-term use of a Foley catheter.
References 172, 184, 215, 532, 549, 601.

Urinary Retention

Related factors: Moderate prostatic hypertrophy; postsurgical pain*

Audrey M. McLane and Ruth E. McShane

PATIENT GOALS/ EXPECTED OUTCOMES	NURSING INTERVENTIONS/ *SCIENTIFIC RATIONALE*
Reestablish usual voiding pattern as evidenced by the following: Voids every 3 to 4 hours Empties bladder completely	Use 100% silicone catheter for indwelling catheter in immediate postoperative period. Select appropriate catheter size. *Too large of a catheter obstructs seminal ducts and may lead to epididymitis and/or prostatitis; usual size is 16 to 18 French in male patient. French catheter scale: each gradation = ⅓ mm. Too narrow a catheter is difficult to insert and permits retrograde extension of bacteria.*
Uses Credé maneuver to facilitate complete emptying of bladder (with physician approval)	Teach Credé maneuver. Teach patient methods to stimulate voiding: stroke lower abdomen or inner thighs; pour warm water over perineum; run water in sink; tap over symphysis pubis. *Stimulation of primitive reflexes facilitates voiding after removal of catheter.*
Verbalizes understanding of role of prostatic hypertrophy in development of urinary retention	Teach patient/family the pathophysiology of prostatic hypertrophy in relation to urinary retention.

*For the patient with bowel resection.

continued.

Urinary Retention—cont'd

PATIENT GOALS/ EXPECTED OUTCOMES	NURSING INTERVENTIONS/ SCIENTIFIC RATIONALE
Develop/adhere to health practices to prevent urinary infection as evidenced by the following:	
Maintains adequate oral intake by taking 8 oz of fluid with meals, between meals, and in early evening	Maintain patient's oral/IV intake at 2000 to 2500 ml unless contraindicated.
Takes superphysiological amounts of vitamin C	Teach patient/family to maintain acid urine (e.g., use superphysiological amounts of ascorbic acid; drink large quantities of cranberry juice). *Keeping urine acidic helps to prevent bladder infections.*
Has no signs or symptoms of infection after removal of catheter as evidenced by the following:	
Reports absence of burning, frequency, and urgency	Monitor patient for signs and symptoms of urinary tract infection.
Urinalysis confirms absence of infection	Obtain daily urinalysis if catheter remains in for more than 48 hours.
	Obtain midstream voided specimen 24 hours after removal of catheter and/or with any signs/symptoms of urinary tract infection (e.g., burning, frequency, urge incontinence).
	Instruct patient/family to call physician if signs/symptoms of infection develop after discharge from hospital.

Urinary Retention—cont'd

PATIENT GOALS/ EXPECTED OUTCOMES	NURSING INTERVENTIONS/ *SCIENTIFIC RATIONALE*
Increase level of activity as evidenced by the following:	
Walks with assistance 4 to 5 times a day	Collaborate with patient to establish increasing activity schedule.
Requests pain medication ½ hour before walking	Provide pain medication ½ hour before walking and initial voiding attempts after removal of catheter.
Stands to void or walks to bathroom after removal of catheter	Have patient stand to void or walk to bathroom after removal of catheter.

References 292, 293, 549, 601.

Ventilation, Inability to Sustain Spontaneous

VENTILATION, INABILITY TO SUSTAIN SPONTANEOUS

Related factor: Imbalance between ventilatory capacity and demand due to decreased ventilatory capacity and/or increased ventilatory demand

Maureen Shekleton and Mi Ja Kim

PATIENT GOALS/ EXPECTED OUTCOMES	NURSING INTERVENTIONS/ SCIENTIFIC RATIONALE
Demonstrate decreased ventilatory demand as evidenced by the following:	

Effective breathing pattern
    Respiratory rate within normal limits
    No accessory muscle use
    Ti/Ttot and Vd/Vt within normal limits
Normal lung compliance
Arterial CO_2 and O_2 concentrations within normal limits
Body temperature within normal limits
Work of breathing (measured) within normal limits
No air trapping at end of expiration (Auto-PEEP)
Normal, clear breath sounds
	Set ventilator to maximize expiratory time (increase inspiratory flow rate or decrease delivered tidal volume). *This setting will decrease occurrence of air trapping or intrinsic PEEP, thus decreasing WOB.*
	Avoid excessive carbohydrate caloric intake.
	Monitor body temperature and treat fever.
	Maintain infection control procedures.
	    Decreased metabolic demands will decrease the ventilatory workload.
	Provide calm, quiet, and comfortable environment.
	Teach relaxation techniques.
	Monitor acid/base status of body fluids and treat alterations.
	    Anxiety, stress, hypoxemia, and acidosis increase respiratory drive, thus increasing ventilatory demand and WOB. Avoiding these conditions decreases demand and WOB.
	Maintain airway patency and clearance by checking size of endotracheal tube and suctioning airway prn. *Decreased air flow resistance minimizes WOB.*

PEEP, positive-end expiratory pressure; *WOB*, work of breathing; *ROM*, range of motion; *Ti*, inspiratory time; *Ttot*, total respiratory time; *Vd*, dead space; *Vt*, tidal volume.

Ventilation, Inability to Sustain Spontaneous—cont'd

PATIENT GOALS/ EXPECTED OUTCOMES	NURSING INTERVENTIONS/ SCIENTIFIC RATIONALE
	Schedule physical activities and exercise routines, as tolerated: up to chair, ambulate, assist with hygiene, and active and passive ROM and bed exercise. *Prevent muscle deconditioning and provide patient with diversionary activities. Muscle deconditioning will contribute to increased ventilatory demand. Diversion helps decrease anxiety.*
Achieve optimal ventilatory capability as evidenced by the following:	
Maximal inspiratory and expiratory pressures within normal limits	Assess nutritional status. Correct nutritional deficits. *Optimal muscle performance depends on adequate supply of nutrients for energy production and protein for muscle tissue repair. In addition, malnutrition blunts respiratory drive.*
Tidal volume and vital capacity within normal limits	
Respiratory rate within normal limits	
	Position to allow maximal thoracic excursion. *Allow diaphragm to contract from optimum length for maximum contractility.*
	Monitor acid/base status of body fluids and correct alterations. *Alkalosis blunts respiratory drive.*
	Monitor effects of sedative agents. *Sedatives can blunt respiratory drive.*

continued.

PATIENT GOALS/ EXPECTED OUTCOMES	NURSING INTERVENTIONS/ *SCIENTIFIC RATIONALE*
	Promote normal rest/sleep patterns. Pace activities to allow rest periods. *Rest allows energy reserves to be replenished. Sleep deprivation blunts respiratory drive.* Provide mechanical ventilatory support at a level that provides rest of respiratory muscles. Use appropriate settings. Apply appropriate mode of ventilation. *Rest is only specific treatment for muscle fatigue. Maximal rest allows complete recovery from fatigue. Improper ventilator settings, type, and cycling and high resistance valves and circuitry add to workload and prevent complete rest and recovery of muscle function.* Provide inspiratory muscle training, if appropriate. *Increase strength and endurance and prevent further deconditioning of respiratory muscles.*

References 48, 197, 351, 528, 584.

Ventilatory Weaning Response, Dysfunctional

Related factors: Physiological and psychological readiness to wean from mechanical ventilation

Maureen Shekleton and Mi Ja Kim

PATIENT GOALS/ EXPECTED OUTCOMES	NURSING INTERVENTIONS/ SCIENTIFIC RATIONALE
Achieve stable, optimal physiological status as evidenced by the following:	
Alert and rested appearance	Assess and monitor respiratory, hemodynamic, metabolic, hydration, and CNS parameters.
Heart rate and rhythm, blood pressure, respiratory rate, tidal volume, electrolytes (especially K^+, Mg^{++}, PO_4), Hgb, Hct, arterial blood gases, weaning parameters, serum albumin, and albumin/globulin ratio within normal limits	Maintain proper ventilator settings. *Inappropriate settings can increase ventilatory workload and predispose respiratory muscles to fatigue. Appropriate settings promote rest of respiratory muscles.*
Balanced intake and output	Encourage adequate intake of food and fluids.
Weight stable and within target ideal body weight range	Provide nutritional supplementation as needed.
No complaints of dyspnea	Obtain nutritional consultation.
Effective airway clearance; normal, clear breath sounds; minimal secretions	*Normal muscle performance and adequate energy supply depend on matching nutritional requirements to metabolic needs.*
Effective breathing pattern— complete, equal, bilateral chest excursion and no paradoxical breathing	Promote normal rest/sleep patterns. Allow 1- to 2-hour rest periods before weaning trial. *Rest is necessary to replenish depleted energy reserves and promote optimal muscle and organ system function.*
No complaints of pain	Maintain airway patency and clearance.
	Check size of endotracheal tube.
	Check placement of endotracheal tube.
	Suction airway prn before weaning trial

continued.

PATIENT GOALS/ EXPECTED OUTCOMES	NURSING INTERVENTIONS/ *SCIENTIFIC RATIONALE*

	Decreased air flow resistance minimizes the work of breathing.
	Position with head elevated, back straight from waist (in chair, on side of bed, in high Fowler's). *Maximal thoracic excursion allows increased lung volumes, thus increasing ventilation to participate in gas exchange.*
	Promote comfort and relieve pain.
	  Teach relaxation techniques.
	  Provide diversionary activities.
	  Administer analgesic medication.
	  Discomfort and pain increase anxiety and cause ineffective breathing patterns, such as "splinted" respiration or rapid, shallow breathing that increases dead space.

Demonstrate feelings of control and independence and minimal anxiety as evidenced by the following:
Calm, relaxed appearance
Verbalizes understanding of weaning plans
States satisfaction with answers to questions
Expresses minimal feelings of anxiety and powerlessness
	Discuss weaning plan with patient and significant others.
	  Explain procedures to be followed.
	  Solicit and answer questions.
	  Reassure that continuous monitoring will occur during weaning trial.
	  Reassure that multiple weaning trials are normal and expected.

Ventilatory Weaning Response, Dysfunctional—cont'd

PATIENT GOALS/ EXPECTED OUTCOMES	NURSING INTERVENTIONS/ *SCIENTIFIC RATIONALE*
	Explain alarm systems and all safety measures being implemented. *Increased understanding will promote cooperation with plan and increase belief in ability and motivation to succeed, as well as decrease anxiety about weaning trial.*
During weaning trial: tolerate decreased ventilatory rate or level of pressure support or total discontinuation of mechanical ventilatory support as evidenced by the following: Stable breathing pattern with minimal initial increase in respiratory rate and decrease in tidal volume. Stable blood pressure, heart rate, and rhythm Stable arterial blood gas levels Breath sounds remain clear Quiet, comfortable breathing without complaints of dyspnea, fatigue, or excessive warmth or discomfort Skin of face and peripheral extremities remains warm and dry and pink in color	Communicate confidence in patient's readiness and ability to wean. Provide comfortable and calm environment with appropriate lighting, temperature, and support persons. *These actions increase patient's level of confidence in self and decreases anxiety level.* Implement collaboratively developed individualized weaning plan that includes goals, methods, and time frames. *Use of a plan that incorporates weaning protocols agreed on by all health-care team members promotes consistency of approach and increases weaning success rate.*

continued.

Ventilatory Weaning Response, Dysfunctional—cont'd

PATIENT GOALS/ EXPECTED OUTCOMES	NURSING INTERVENTIONS/ SCIENTIFIC RATIONALE
	Remain with patient and monitor status continuously during weaning trial. *Promote safety, because change can occur rapidly and may require immediate intervention.*
	Suction airway prn during weaning trial. *Maintain airway potency and decrease resistance to air flow, thus minimizing work of breathing.*
	Provide fan at bedside. *Sensation of coolness and blowing air lessens feelings of shortness of breath.*
	Communicate progress in achieving weaning goals to patient and significant others as weaning process continues. *Positive feedback increases motivation.*

References 92, 277, 300, 335, 336, 353.

Violence, High Risk for: Self-Directed or Directed at Others

Risk factor: Antisocial character*

Gertrude K. McFarland and Lorna A. Larson

PATIENT GOALS/ EXPECTED OUTCOMES	NURSING INTERVENTIONS/ *SCIENTIFIC RATIONALE*
Experience a reduced potential for violence as evidenced by the following:	
Verbalizes less aggression	Monitor patient for the following:
Decreases frequency of assaultive behavior	Verbal aggression (e.g., angry shouting)
Verbalizes anger appropriately	Physical aggression against self (e.g., suicidal gestures)
Demonstrates positive regard for others	Perceptions of self and environment
Controls own behavior	Value system in which violence is viewed as acceptable response
Refrains from harming self or others	Preconceived plan for harming self or others
Identifies therapeutic resources available to help change behavior	Strong interest in and/or availability of weapons
Demonstrates constructive coping skills in dealing with stress and frustration	Ideas of persecution
	Short attention span
	Low tolerance to frustration
	Early interventions in the preceding factors can prevent a violent episode.
	Variations in perception. *If the variation in perception is disturbing to the individual, violence may be used to force greater congruence of perceptions.*
	Effects of drugs/medications. *A side effect of drugs/medications can be violence.*

---

*For the patient with antisocial personality disorder. *continued.*

Violence, High Risk for: Self-Directed or Directed at Others—cont'd

PATIENT GOALS/ EXPECTED OUTCOMES	NURSING INTERVENTIONS/ SCIENTIFIC RATIONALE
	Determine additional risk factors:
	History or physical aggression against objects/others
	History of life stressors
	History of family violence
	History of parental discipline patterns as a child. *The more abusive, the greater the potential for violence.*
	A past history of any of the preceding additional risk factors predisposes an individual to coping with life or in obtaining a desired end through the use of violence.
	Create ward environment that is light, open, and uncrowded with a low noise level and adequate staffing *so that the patient can feel safe and know that the staff can control any violence that occurs. The low noise level decreases arousal/ agitation, which can lead to violence.*
	Avoid a tone of voice that suggests nagging, pessimism, indifference, or hostility.
	Do not respond to abusive language with abusive language.
	Avoid direct confrontation.
	Patients respond to these staff behaviors defensively (sometimes violently) because they are perceived as a threat to the self.

Violence, High Risk for: Self-Directed or Directed at Others—cont'd

PATIENT GOALS/ EXPECTED OUTCOMES	NURSING INTERVENTIONS/ SCIENTIFIC RATIONALE
	Avoid extensive eye-to-eye contact, especially when anger is intensifying. *Eye contact can be perceived as an assertion of dominance over the individual and can lead to defensive violence.*
	Always respond to questions asked by patient. *This increases the patient's feeling of worth and decreases the need for violence to obtain what is desired.*
	Establish hospital unit norm against physical harm to self or others with set sanctions for infractions. *The expectation that violence will not be tolerated decreases violence.*
	Provide opportunities for aerobic exercises 3 to 7 times a week. *This uses a socially acceptable way of expressing angry feelings, decreasing agitation, and maintaining health.*
	Provide one-to-one supportive counseling *to identify coping mechanisms and to recognize consequences of violent behavior.*
	Provide nurse-group psychotherapy *to eliminate interpersonal dysfunctions, develop better communication skills, and foster socialization.*

continued.

Violence, High Risk for: Self-Directed or Directed at Others—cont'd

PATIENT GOALS/ EXPECTED OUTCOMES	NURSING INTERVENTIONS/ *SCIENTIFIC RATIONALE*
	Provide positive reinforcement of behaviors that help to decrease/control violent behavior, *because this rewards the patient's attempts to use socially acceptable behaviors.* Recommend or provide family therapy *to resolve family issues/conflicts and to empower the family in coping with and establishing sanctions for the violent family member.* Teach patient the following: 　About accountability for own behavior (e.g., if patient breaks something, he/she must pay for it or work to pay it off; if injury to self or others, he/she must provide restitution within limits of program) 　To recognize impending violence and to assume responsibility for aborting the violence 　To learn alternate coping mechanisms, such as negotiating skills, socially acceptable ways of expressing feelings of anger and hostility, and/or stress-reducing/relaxation skills *Alternative coping mechanisms for stress or perceived threats decrease the need to use violence for coping.*

References 91, 312, 489, 502, 567, 638.

To be developed diagnostic concepts and definitions*

*Handout, Tenth conference for classification of nursing diagnoses, San Diego, Calif, 1992.

1. **Activity Level, Excessive**

   Energy that is being displayed to a level that is beyond the usual measure or proportion. An above "relative normal" state of energy expenditure is a change or a difference that creates stress, which in turn results in needs.

2. **Altered Family Processes: Addictive Behavior (Individual and Family)**

   The state in which the psychosocial, spiritual, and physiological functions of a family unit are chronically disorganized, leading to conflict, denial of problems, resistance to change, ineffective problem solving, and a series of self-perpetuating crises.

3. **Altered Parent/Infant Attachment**

   Disruption of the interactive process between parent/significant other and infant that fosters the development of a protective and nurturing reciprocal relationship.

4. **Confusion, Acute**

   The abrupt onset of a cluster of global, transient changes and disturbances in attention, cognition, psychomotor activity, level of consciousness, and/or sleep-wake cycle.

5. **Confusion, Chronic**

   An irreversible, long-standing, and/or progressive deterioration of intellect and personality characterized by decreased ability to interpret environmental stimuli, decreased capacity for intellectual thought processes, and manifested by disturbances of memory, orientation, and behavior.

6. **Decisional Conflict, Family: Required**

   Identifies the disequilibrium that occurs among and within family members when the family unit must reach a consensus within a specific time frame. Time constraints and associated ethical and/or value-laden consequences may prompt crisis and uncertainty, further blocking the decision-making process.

7. **Decreased Adaptive Capacity, Intracranial**

   A clinical state in which intracranial fluid dynamic mechanisms that normally compensate for increases in intracranial volumes are compromised, resulting in repeated disproportionate increases in intracranial pressure (ICP) over baseline in response to a variety of noxious and non-noxious stimuli.

8. **High Risk for Disproportionate Increase in Intracranial Pressure**

   A clinical state in which a person with baseline increased ICP is at risk for developing disproportionately large and sustained increases over baseline ICP (greater than 10 mm

Hg over baseline for more than 5 minutes) in response to external stimuli.

9. **High Risk for Loneliness**
   A subjective state in which an individual is at risk of experiencing vague dysphoria.

10. **High Risk for Impaired Skin Integrity: Pressure Ulcer**
    A state in which the individual's skin is at risk of being adversely affected.

11. **Idiopathic Fecal Incontinence**
    A change in an individual's pattern of elimination characterized by a loss of ability to voluntarily control the passage of feces/gas and occasional/frequent loss of normal stool.

12. **Impaired Feeding Drive**
    A state in which a nutritionally sound patient has difficulty returning to normal eating patterns during illness or recovery from illness.

13. **Impaired Memory**
    The state in which an individual experiences an inability to remember or recall bits of information or behavioral skills. Impaired memory may be attributed to pathophysiological or situational causes that are either temporary or permanent.

14. **Ineffective Coping (Communities)**
    A pattern of community activities for adaptation and problem solving that is unsatisfactory for meeting the demands or needs of the community.

15. **Ineffective Management of Therapeutic Regimen (Families)**
    A pattern of regulating and integrating into family processes a program for treatment of illness and the sequelae of illness that is unsatisfactory for meeting specific health goals.

16. **Labor Pain**
    A subjective measure of an unpleasant sensation that lasts the duration of a contraction and may linger between contractions. The feeling subsides with delivery of the infant.

17. **Potential for Enhanced Coping (Communities)**
    A pattern of community activities for adaptation and problem solving that is satisfactory for meeting the demands or needs of the community but can be improved for management of current and future problems/stressors.

18. **Potential for Enhanced Spiritual Well-Being**
    The process of an individual's developing/unfolding of mystery through harmonious interconnectedness that springs from inner strengths.

19. **Spasticity**

    The state in which an individual with an upper motor neuron injury experiences increased muscle tone and abnormal reflexes in response to internal or external stimuli that interfere with functional abilities such as mobility, hygiene, eating, dressing, and toileting.

20. **Terminal Illness Response**

    That time when a terminal illness develops or is diagnosed, and a patient tries to deal with the pending, permanent separation from loved ones, possessions, and his/her own body. If a patient is unconscious, the family, significant other, or caregiver may experience the phenomena alone.

REFERENCES

1. Aasen N: Interventions to facilitate personal control, *J Gerontol Nurs* 13(6):21, 1987.
2. Abernathy E: Biological response modifiers, *Am J Nurs* 87(4):458, 1987.
3. Abruzzese R, ed: The integumentary system, *Top Clin Nurs* 5(2), 1983.
4. Adam K: Dietary habits and sleep after bedtime food drinks, *Sleep* 3(1):47, 1980.
5. Aquilera D, Messick L: *Crisis intervention,* St Louis, 1990, Mosby–Year Book.
6. Aistars J: Fatigue in the cancer patient: a conceptual approach to a clinical problem, *Oncol Nurs Forum* 14(6):25, 1987.
7. Allan JD: Exercise program. In Bulechek GM, McCloskey JC, eds: *Nursing interventions: essential nursing treatments,* ed 2, Philadelphia, 1992, WB Saunders.
8. Allan JD, Hall BA: Between diagnosis and death: the case for studying grief before death, *Arch Psychiatric Nurs* 2(1):30, 1988.
9. Alterescu KB, Alteresen V: The treatment of pressure sores. In Catania PN, Rosner MM, eds: *Home health care practice,* Palo Alto, Calif, 1986, Health Markets Research.
10. Alterescu V: Theoretical foundations for an approach to fecal incontinence, *J Enterostom Ther* 13:44, 1986.
11. Alteri C: The patient with myocardial infarction: rest prescriptions for activities of daily living, *Heart Lung* 13:4, 1984.
11a. American Academy of Pediatrics Committee on Nutrition: Human milk banking, *Ped* 65:854, 1980b.
12. American Association of Critical-Care Nurses: *AACN outcome standards for nursing care of the critically ill,* Calif, 1990, The Association.
13. American Thoracic Society: Research priorities in respiratory nursing, *Am Rev Respir Dis* 142:1459, 1990.
14. American Thoracic Society: Standards for the diagnosis and care of patients with chronic obstructive pulmonary disease (COPD) and asthma, *Am Rev Respir Dis* 136:225, 1987.
15. American Thoracic Society: Standards of nursing care for adult patients with pulmonary dysfunction, *Am Rev Respir Dis* 143:231, 1991.
16. Ammerman RT: Etiological models of child maltreatment: a behavioral perspective, *Behavior Modif* 14:230, 1990.

366

17. Andersen AN and others: Suppressed prolactin but normal neuro-physin levels in cigarette smoking breast-feeding women, *Clin Endocrinol* 17:363, 1962.

17a. Anderson GH and Hrboticky N: Approaches to assessing the dietary component of the diet-behavior connection, *Nutr Rev Suppl*, pp 42-50, May 1986.

18. Anderson JM, Ellert H: Managing chronic illness in the family: women as caretakers, *J Adv Nurs* 14:735, 1989.

19. Anderson JZ, White GD: An empirical investigation of interaction and relationship patterns in functional and dysfunctional nuclear families and stepfamilies, *Fam Process* 25:407, 1986.

20. Andreoli K and others: *Comprehensive cardiac care,* ed 6, St Louis, 1987, Mosby–Year Book.

21. Andrews HA: Overview of the role function mode. In Roy SR, Andrews A, eds: *The Roy Adaptation Model,* Norwalk, Conn, 1991, Appleton & Lange.

22. Annon JS: *Behavioral treatment of sexual problems: brief therapy,* Hagerstown, Md, 1976, Harper & Row.

23. Antman EM: Digitalis toxicity, *Modern Concepts of Cardiovascular Disease* 55(6):26, 1986.

24. Antonucci TC, Jackson JS: Physical health and self-esteem, *Family Commun Health* 6(2):1, 1983.

25. Antonucci TC, Peggs JF, Marquez JT: The relationship between self-esteem and physical health in a family practice population, *Family Pract Res J* 9(1):65, 1989.

26. Archbold PG and others: Mutuality and preparedness as predictors of caregiver role strain, *Res Nurs Health* 3:375, 1990.

27. Aroian KJ: A model of psychological adaptation to migration and resettlement, *Nurs Res* 39(1):5, 1990.

28. Aronson TA: A critical review of psychotherapeutic treatments of the borderline personality, *J Nerv Ment Dis* 177(9):511, 1989.

29. Auerbach K: Assisting the employed breastfeeding mother, *J Nurse Midwifery* 35(1):26, 1990.

30. Augustine S: Hypothermia therapy in the postanesthesia unit: a review, *J Post Anesth Nurs* 5(4):254, 1990.

31. Autry D, Lauzon F, Holliday P: The voiding record: an aid in decreasing incontinence, *Geriatr Nurs* 5(1):22, 1984.

32. Axelsson K, Norberg A, Asplund K: Relearning to eat late after a stroke by systematic nursing intervention: a case report, *J Adv Nurs* 11:553, 1986.

33. Azar ST, Siegel BK: Behavioral treatment of child abuse: a developmental perspective, *Behavior Modif* 14:279, 1990.

34. Baggs JG, Karch AM: Sexual counseling of women with coronary heart disease, *Heart Lung* 16(2):154, 1987.

35. Baker S, O'Neill B, Karpf R: *The injury fact book,* Lexington, Mass, 1984, DC Heath & Co.

36. Baker WL, Smith SL: Pulmonary aspiration and tube feedings: nursing implications, *Focus Crit Care* 11(2):25, 1984.

37. Barlow DH: Long-term outcome for patients with panic disorder treated with cognitive behavioral therapy, *J Clin Psychiatry* 51(A):17, 1990.

38. Barnes S: Patient/family education for the patient with pressure necrosis, *Nurs Clin North Am* 22(2):463, 1987.

39. Beard M, Enlow C, Owen J: Activity therapy as a reconstructive plan on the social competence of chronic hospitalized patients, *J Psychiatr Nurs Ment Health Serv* 16:33, 1978.

40. Beaver B: Health education and the patient with peripheral vascular disease, *Nurs Clin North Am* 21(2):265, 1986.

41. Beck AT: *Cognitive therapy of personality disorders,* New York, 1990, Guilford Press.

42. Becker PM, Jamieson AO: Common sleep disorders in the elderly: diagnosis and treatment, *Geriatrics* 47(3):41, 1992.

43. Bednar RI, Wells MG, Peterson SR: *Self-esteem: paradoxes and innovations in clinical theory and practice,* Washington, DC, 1989, American Psychological Association.

44. Beglinger JE: Coping tasks in critical care, *Dimens Crit Care Nurs* 2(2):80, 1983.

45. Belgrave FZ: Psychosocial predictors of adjustment to disability in African Americans, *J Rehabil* 57(1):37, 1991.

46. Bell L, Shronts E: Nutritional support in respiratory failure, *Nutritional Support in Critical Care,* Rockville, Md, 1987, Aspen.

47. Bellemare F, Grassino A: Force reserve of the diaphragm in patients with chronic obstructive pulmonary disease, *J Appl Physiol* 55:8, 1983.

48. Benotti PN, Bistrian B: Metabolic and nutritional aspects of weaning from mechanical ventilation, *Crit Care Med* 17:181, 1989.

49. Bergstrom N and others: The Braden scale for predicting pressure sore risk, *Nurs Res* 36(4):205, 1987.

50. Biaggio MK: Clinical dimensions of anger management, *Am J Psychother* 41:417, 1987.

51. Bigner JJ: *Parent-child relations: an introduction to parenting,* New York, 1989, Macmillan.

52. Bixler EO, Vela-Bueno A: Correlates of normal sleep, *Psychiatr Ann* 17(7):437, 1987.

53. Blank C, Irwin GH: Peripheral vascular disorders, *Nurs Clin North Am* 25(4):777, 1990.

54. Bobel L: Nutritional implications in the patient with pressure sores, *Nurs Clin North Am* 22(2):379, 1987.

55. Bodkin WL and Hansen BC: Nutritional studies in nursing, *Ann Rev Nurs Res* 9:203, 1991.

56. Bonheur B, Young SW: Exercise as a health-promoting lifestyle choice, *Appl Nurs Res* 4(1):2, 1991.

57. Bonica JJ: The need for a taxonomy of pain, *Pain* 6(3):247, 1979.

58. Boozer M, Craven R: Nursing care of the patient with chronic occlusive peripheral artery disease, *Cardiovasc Nurs* 15(4):13, 1981.

59. Bostwick J, Wendelmass ST: Normal saline instillation as part of the suctioning procedure: effects on PaO_2 and amount of secretions, *Heart Lung* 16:532, 1987.

60. Botsford KB and others: Gram-negative bacilli in human milk feedings: quantitation and clinical consequences for premature infants, *J Pediatr* 109:707, 1987.

61. Boutell KA, Bozett FW: Nurses' assessment of patients' spirituality: continuing education implications, *J Contin Educ Nurs* 21(4):172, 1990.

62. Bowers BJ: Intergenerational caregiving: adult caregivers and their aging parents, *Adv Nurs Sci* 9(2):20, 1987.

368

63. Bowers JE: Coping, family, potential for growth. In McFarland GK, Thomas MD: *Psychiatric mental health nursing: application of the nursing process,* Philadelphia, 1991, JB Lippincott.

64. Bowers S, Marshall L: Severe head injury: current treatment and research, *J Neurosurg Nurs* 14:210, 1982.

65. Boynton P: Health maintenance alteration: a nursing diagnosis of the elderly, *Clin Nurs Spec* 3(1):5, 1989.

66. Brager B, Yasko J: *Stomatitis, in care of the client receiving chemotherapy,* Reston, Va, 1984, Reston Publishing.

67. Brandt PA, Weinert C: The PRQ: a social support measure, *Nurs Res* 30:277, 1981.

68. Braunwald E: Regulation of the circulation, *N Engl J Med* 290:1124, 1974.

69. Breitenstine NL: Validation of diagnostic cues of body image disturbance in clients who undergo orthopedic internal implant surgery. In Carroll-Johnson RM, ed: *Classification of nursing diagnoses: proceedings of the eighth conference,* Philadelphia, 1989, JB Lippincott.

70. Brennan-Behn M and others: Lipid loss during continuous nasogastric infusion of mother's milk: a comparison of two methods. (Unpublished data).

71. Breslin EH, Lery MJ: Prevention and treatment of aspiration pneumonitis secondary to massive gastric aspiration, *Crit Care Q* 73, 1983.

71a. Brewerton TD, Hefferman MM, Rosenthal NE: Psychiatric aspects of the relationship between eating and mood, *Nutr Rev Suppl* 78, May 1986.

72. Breznitz S: The seven kinds of denial. In Breznitz S, ed: *The denial of stress,* New York, 1983, International Universities Press.

73. Bridges W: *Transitions—making sense of life's changes,* Reading, Mass, 1980, Addison-Wesley.

74. Brodaty H, Gresham M: Effect of training programme to reduce stress in careers of patients with dementia, *BMJ* 299(6712):1375, 1989.

75. Brophy LR, Sharp EJ: Physical symptoms of combination biotherapy: a quality of life issue, *Oncol Nurs Forum* 18(1):25, 1991.

76. Bruce J, Grove S: Fever: pathology and treatment, *Crit Care Nurs* 12(1):40, 1992.

77. Bruno P: Skin problems. In Carnevali DL, Patrick M, eds: *Nursing management for the elderly,* ed 2, Philadelphia, 1986, JB Lippincott.

78. Bruss C: Nursing diagnosis of hopelessness, *J Psychosoc Nurs Ment Health Serv* 26:28, 1988.

79. Buck MH: The personal self. In Roy SC, Andrews A: *The Roy adapation model,* Norwalk, Conn, 1991, Appleton & Lange.

80. Bulechek GM, McCloskey JC, eds: *Nursing interventions: essential nursing treatments,* ed 2, Philadelphia, 1992, WB Saunders.

80a. Bulechek GM, McCloskey JC, eds: *Nursing interventions: treatments for nursing diagnoses,* Philadelphia, 1985, WB Saunders.

81. Bull MJ: Factors influencing family caregiver burden and health, *West J Nurs Res* 12(6):758, 1990.

82. Bunting SM: Stress on caregivers of the elderly, *Adv Nurs Sci* 11(2):63, 1990.

83. Burckhardt CS: Coping strategies of the chronically ill, *Nurs Clin North Am* 22(3):543, 1987.

84. Burgess AW: *Psychiatric nursing in the hospital and the community,* Norwalk, Conn, 1990, Appleton & Lange.

85. Burgess AW, Holstrom LL: Rape: sexual disruption and recovery, *Am J Orthopsychiatry* 49:648, 1979.

85a. Burgess AW, Holstrom LL: Rape trauma syndrome, *Am J Psychiatry* 131:981, 1974.

86. Burgess AW and others: HIV testing of sexual assault populations: ethical and legal issues, *J Emerg Nurs* 16(5):331, 1990.

87. Burgio K: A continence clinic: using biofeedback and other behavioral methods for the treatment of urinary incontinence. Paper presentation, CNR Conference: Nursing research: integration into the social structure, San Diego, 1985.

88. Burgio KL, Whitehead WE, Engel BT: Urinary incontinence in the elderly: bladder-sphincter biofeedback and toilet skills training, *Ann Intern Med* 104:507, 1984.

89. Burish TG, Snyder SL, Jenkins RA: Preparing patients for cancer chemotherapy: effect of coping preparation and relaxation interventions, *J Consult Clin Psychol* 59(4):518, 1991.

90. Burke LE: Cardiovascular disturbances and sexuality. In Fogel CI, Lauver D: *Sexual health promotion,* Philadelphia, 1990, WB Saunders.

91. Cahill C and others: Inpatient management of violent behavior: nursing prevention and intervention, *Issues Men Health Nurs* 12:239, 1991.

92. Calhoun CJ, Specht NL: Standardizing the weaning process, *AACN Clinic Issues Crit Care Nurs* 2(3):398, 1991.

93. Call JG, Davis LL: The effect of hardiness on coping strategies and adjustment to illness in chronically ill individuals, *Appl Nurs Res* 2(4):187, 1989.

94. Callahan J: Compartment syndrome, *Orthop Nurs* 4(4):11, 1985.

95. Carlson SL: Altered health maintenance. In McFarland GK, McFarlane EA: *Nursing diagnosis and intervention,* St Louis, 1989, Mosby–Year Book.

96. Camp-Sorrell D: Controlling adverse effects of chemotherapy, *Nursing* 21(4):34, 1991.

97. Carmen EH, Rieker PP: A psychosocial model of the victim-to-patient process, *Psychiatr Clin North Am* 12(2):431, 1989.

98. Carpenito LJ: *Nursing diagnosis: application to clinical practice,* ed 4, New York, 1992, JB Lippincott.

99. Carpenito LJ: Nursing diagnosis in critical care: impact on practice and outcomes, *Heart Lung* 16:595, 1987.

100. Carpenter KD: Recognizing the many faces of fear, *Nurs Life* 6(4):29, 1986.

101. Carroll SM: *Clinical validation study of hypothermia: identification of defining characteristics,* unpublished manuscript.

102. Casperson CJ, Powell KE, Christenson GM: Physical activity, exercise and physical fitness: definitions and distinctions for health-related research, *Public Health Report* 100:126, 1985.

103. Cavanaugh JA: Overdrive pacing: an approach to terminating ventricular tachycardia, *J Cardiovasc Nurs* 5(3):58, 1991.

104. Chagares R, Jackson B: Sitting easy: how six pressure-relieving devices stack up, *Am J Nurs* 87(2):191, 1987.

105. Champion VL: The relationship of selected variables to breast cancer detection behaviors in women 35 and older, *Oncol Nurs Forum* 18(4):733, 1991.

106. Chernoff R, Dean JA: Medical and nutritional aspects of intractable diarrhea, *J Am Diet Assoc* 76:161, 1980.

107. Chopra S and others: Effects of hydration and physical therapy on tracheal transport velocity, *Am Rev Respir Dis* 115:1009, 1977.

108. Christman NJ, Kirchoff KT, Oakley MG: Concrete objective information. In Bulechek GM, McCloskey JC, eds: *Nursing interventions: essential nursing treatment*, ed 2, Philadelphia, 1992, WB Saunders.

109. Churella HR, Bachhuber WL, MacLean WC: Survey: methods of feeding low-birth weight infants, *Pediatrics* 76:243, 1985.

110. Clay E: Habit retraining: a tested method to regain urinary control, *Geriatr Nurs* 1:252, 1980.

111. Clay K, Stirn M: Documentation of discharge teaching of patients who have had hip surgery, *Orthop Nurs* 5(6):22, 1986.

112. Clinton P, Eland JA: Pain. In Maas M, Buckwalter KC, Hardy M, eds: *Nursing diagnoses and interventions for the elderly,* Redwood City, Calif, 1991, Addison-Wesley.

113. Clubb RL: Chronic sorrow: adaptation patterns of parents with chronically ill children, *Pediatr Nurs* 17:461, 1991.

114. Cohen F: Immunologic impairment, infection and AIDS in the aging patient, *Crit Care Nurse Q* 12(1):38, 1989.

115. Cohn J: Vasodilator therapy: implications in acute myocardial infarction and congestive heart failure, *Am Heart J* 49:45, 1982.

116. Cohn JN and others: Effect of vasodilator therapy on mortality in chronic congestive heart failure, *N Engl J Nurs* 47, 1986.

117. Colburn L: Preventing pressure ulcers, *Nursing* 20(12):60, 1990.

118. Conn L, Lion J: Self-mutilation: a review, *Psychiatr Med* 1(1):21, 1983.

119. Conn VS, Taylor SG, Kelley S: Medication regimen complexity and adherence among older adults, *Image: J Nurs Sch* 23(4):231, 1991.

120. Cook AS, Oltjenbruns KA: *Dying and grieving,* New York, 1989, Holt, Rinehart & Winston.

121. Cooney NL and others: Matching alcoholics to coping skills or interactional therapies: two-year follow-up results, *J Consult Clin Psychol* 59(4):598, 1991.

122. Cooper D: Pressure ulcers: unpublished research, 1976-1986, *Nurs Clin North Am* 22(2):475, 1987.

123. Coopersmith S: *The antecedents of self-esteem,* San Francisco, 1967, WH Freeman.

124. Cornwell CJ, Schmitt MH: Perceived health status, self-esteem, and body image in women with rheumatoid arthritis or systemic lupus erythematosus, *Res Nurs Health* 13:99, 1990.

125. Cousins N: *The healing heart,* New York, 1983, WW Norton & Co.

126. Cox CL: The health self-determinism index, *Nurs Res* 34(3):177, 1985.

127. Cox CL, Miller EH, Mull CS: Motivation in health behavior: measurement, antecedents, and correlates, *Adv Nurs Sci* 9(4):1, 1987.

128. Craig H: Accuracy of indirect measures of medication compliance in hypertension, *Res Nurs Health* 8:61, 1985.

129. Creason NS and others: Validating the diagnosis of impaired physical mobility, *Nurs Clin North Am* 20:669, 1985.

130. Crist JK: Weight management. In Bulechek GM, McCloskey JC, eds: *Nursing interventions: essential nursing treatments,* ed 2, Philadelphia, 1992 WB Saunders.

131. Crouch MA, Straub V: Enhancement of self-esteem in adults, *Fam Community Health* 6(2):67, 1983.

132. Crowther D: Metacommunications: a missed opportunity, *J Psychosoc Nurs Ment Health Serv* 29:13, 1991.

133. Crumbaugh JC, Maholick LT: *Purpose in life test.* Available from Psychometric Affiliates, PO Box 3167, Munster, Ind 46231.

134. Cunha B, Tu R: Fever in the neurosurgical patient, *Heart Lung* 17(6):608, 1988.

135. Curry LC, Stone JG: The grief process: a preparation for death, *Clinical Nurse Specialist* 5(1):17, 1991.

136. Cuzzell JZ, Willey T: Pressure relief perennials, *Am J Nurs* 87(9):1157, 1987.

137. Czurylo K, Kim MJ: Infection, potential for. In Kim MJ, McFarland GK, McLane AM: *Pocket guide to nursing diagnoses,* ed 3, St Louis, 1989, Mosby–Year Book.

138. Daeffler R: Oral hygiene measures for patients with cancer, I, *Cancer Nurs* 3(5):347, 1980.

139. Daeffler R: Oral hygiene measures for patients with cancer, II, *Cancer Nurs* 3(6):427, 1980.

140. Daeffler R: Oral hygiene measures for patients with cancer, III, *Cancer Nurs* 4(1):29, 1981.

141. Davis M, Eshelman ER, McKay M: *The relaxation and stress reduction workbook,* Oakland, Calif, 1982, New Harbinger.

142. DeCarlo JJ, Mann WC: The effectiveness of verbal versus activity groups in improving self-perceptions of interpersonal communication skills, *Am J Occup Ther* 39(1):20, 1985.

143. DeCarvalho M, Robertson S, Klaus MH: Does the duration and frequency of early breastfeeding affect nipple pain? *Birth* 11(2):81, 1984.

144. DeChenne TK: Boredom as a clinical issue, *Psychotherapy* 25:71, 1988.

145. Dexter W: Hypothermia, *Post Graduate Medicine* 88(8):55, 1990.

146. Dickey JW: Stasis ulcers: the role of compliances in healing, *South Med J* 84(5):557, 1991.

147. Price M, DiIorio M: Swallowing: a practice guide, *Am J Nurs* 90(7):42, 1990.

148. DiNisi J and others: Comparison of cardiovascular responses to noise during waking and sleeping in humans, *Sleep* 13(2):108, 1990.

149. Dittmar S: *Rehabilitation nursing—process and application,* St Louis, 1989, Mosby–Year Book.

150. Doenges ME, Moorhouse M, Geissler AC: *Nursing care plans—guidelines for planning patient care,* ed 2, Philadelphia, 1989, FA Davis.

151. Doenges ME, Townsend MC, Moorhouse MF: *Psychiatric care plans—guidelines for client care,* Philadelphia, 1989, FA Davis.

152. Donahue W and others: Long-term mechanical ventilation guidelines for management in the home and at alternate community sites, *Chest* 90(1):1S, 1986.

153. Donnelly C: Ending the torment, *Nurs Times* 87(11):36, 1991.

154. Doyle J: Treatment modalities in peripheral vascular disease, *Nurs Clin North Am* 21(2):241, 1986.

155. Dracup K, Brev C: Using nursing research findings to meet the need of grieving spouses, *Nurs Res* 27:212, 1978.

156. Drew BJ: Cardiac responses. I. Important phenomenon for nursing practice, science, and research, *Heart Lung* 18(1), 1989.

157. Duffy ME: Determinants of health promotion, *Nurs Res* 37(6):358, 1988.

158. Dusdieker L and others: Prolonged maternal fluid supplementation in breast-feeding, *Pediatrics* 86(5):737, 1990.

159. Eastwood HDH, Warrell R: Urinary incontinence in the elderly female: prediction in diagnosis and outcome of management, *Age Ageing* 13:230, 1985.

160. Ellerhorst-Ryan JM: Measuring aspects of spirituality. In Frank-Stromberg, M, ed: *Instruments for clinical nursing research*, Norwalk, Conn, 1988, Appleton & Lange.

161. Elliopoulous C: *Nursing care planning guides for long-term care*, ed 3, Baltimore, Md, 1990, Williams & Wilkins.

162. Elsen J, Blegen M: Social isolation. In Maas M, Buckwalter KC, Hardy M, eds: *Nursing diagnoses and interventions for the elderly*, Philadelphia, 1991, WB Saunders.

163. Emick-Herring B, Wood P: A team approach to neurologically based swallowing disorders, *Rehabil Nurs* 15(3):126, 1990.

164. Epstein NR and others: A system therapy: problem-centered systems therapy of the family. In Wells RA, Giannetti VJ, eds: *Handbook of the brief psychotherapies*, New York, 1990, Plenum Press.

165. Erickson R, Yount S: Effect of aluminized covers on body temperature in patients having abdominal surgery, *Heart Lung* 20(3):255, 1991.

166. Estes NM, Smith-DiJulio K, Heinemann ME: *Nursing diagnosis of the alcoholic person*, St Louis, 1980, Mosby–Year Book.

167. Farrell J: *Illustrated guide to orthopedic nursing*, ed 3, Philadelphia, 1986, JB Lippincott.

168. Favazza A: Why patients mutilate themselves, *Hosp Community Psychiatry* 40(2):137, 1989.

169. Feldman M: The challenge of self-mutilation: a review, *Compr Psychiatry* 29(2):252, 1988.

170. Fellows E, Jocz AM: Getting the upper hand on lower extremity arterial disease, *Nursing* 21(8):34, 1991.

171. Ferran C, Popovich J: Hope: a relevant concept for geriatric psychiatry, *Arch Psychiatr Nurs* 4:124, 1990.

172. Field MS: Urinary incontinence in the elderly: an overview, *J Gerontol Nurs* 5:12, 1979.

173. Figueroa M: A dynamic taxonomy of self-destructive behavior, *Psychotherapy*, 25(2):280, 1988.

174. Finocchiaro DN, Herzfeld ST: Understanding autonomic dysreflexia, *Am J Nurs* 90(9):56, 1990.

175. Fischer K: Adult children of alcholics: implications for the nursing profession, *Nurs Forum* 4:159, 1988.

176. Fisher S: Leaving home: homesickness and the psychological effects of change and transition. In Fisher P, Reason J, eds: *Handbook of life stress, cognition, and health*, New York, 1988, John Wiley & Sons.

177. Fitzmaurice JB: Utilization of cues in judgments of activity intolerance. In McLane AM, ed: *Classification of nursing diagnoses: proceedings of the seventh conference,* St Louis, 1987, Mosby–Year Book.

178. Flannery Jr RB: *Becoming stress resistant: through the project smart program,* New York, 1990, Continuum.

179. Fleury JD: Empowering potential: a theory of wellness motivation, *Nurs Res* 40(5):286, 1991.

180. Forchuck C, Westwell J: Denial, *J Psychosoc Nurs Ment Health Serv* 25(6):9, 1987.

181. Forsyth GL, Delaney KD, Gresham ML: Vying for a winning position: management style of the chronically ill, *Res Nurs Health* 7:181, 1984.

182. Fowler E: Equipment and products used in management and treatment of pressure ulcers, *Nurs Clin North Am* 22(2):449, 1987.

183. Free T and others: A descriptive study of infants and toddlers exposed prenatally to substance abuse, *MCN* 15(4):245, 1990.

184. Freed SL: Urinary incontinence in the elderly, *Hosp Pract* 17:81, 1982.

185. Freeman SK: Inpatient management of a patient with borderline personality disorder: a case study, *Arch Psychiatr Nurs* 2(6):360, 1988.

186. Friedland J: Diversional activity: does it deserve a bad name? *Am J Occup Ther* 42(9):603, 1988.

187. Friedman PA: Chemical intoxication. In Isselbacher KJ and others, eds: *Harrison's principles of internal medicine,* ed 9, New York, 1980, McGraw-Hill.

188. Frye SJ, Lounsbury P: *Cardiac rhythm disorders: an introduction using the nursing process,* Baltimore, 1988, Williams & Wilkins.

189. Gabriel R, Kirschling J: Assessing grief among the bereaved elderly: a review of existing measures, *Hospice J* 5(1):29, 1989.

190. Galvo M: Role of angiotensin-converting enzyme inhibitors in congestive heart failure, *Heart Lung* 19(5):505, 1990.

191. Gara MA, Rosenberg S, Cohen BD: Personal identity and the schizophrenic process: an integration, *Psychiatry* 50(3):267, 1987.

192. Gardner G: Home IV therapy, I, *Nat Intraven Ther Assoc* 9:95, 1986.

192a. Gardner GI: Home IV therapy, II, *Nat Intraven Ther Assoc* 9:193, 1986.

193. Garvin B: Interpersonal communication between nurses and patients, *Annu Rev Nurs Res* 8:213, 1990.

194. Gaynor SE: The long haul: the effects of home care on caregivers. *Image J Nurs Sch* 22(4):208, 1990.

195. Geach B: Pain and coping, *Image J Nurs Sch* 19(1):12, 1987.

196. Geary PA: Stress and social support in the experience of monitoring apneic infants, *Clin Nurse Spec* 3:119, 1989.

197. Geisman LK, Ahrens T: Auto-PEEP: an impediment to weaning in the chronically ventilated patient, *AACN Clin Issues Crit Care Nurs* 2(3):391, 1991.

198. Gettrust K, Ryan S, Engelman DS, eds: *Applied nursing diagnosis: guide for comprehensive care planning,* New York, 1985, John Wiley & Sons.

199. Gilberts R: The evaluation of self-esteem, *Family Community Health* 6(2):29, 1983.

200. Gilts C: Nursing management of mastitis due to breastfeeding, *JOGNN* 14:286, 1985.

201. Given BA, Given CW: Family caregiving for the elderly, *Ann Rev Nurs Res* 9:77, 1991.

202. Glauser F, Polatty R, Sessler C: State of the art: worsening oxygenation in the mechanically ventilated patient—causes, mechanisms and early detection, *Am Rev Respir Dis* 138(2):458, 1988.

203. Glick DF: Home care of patients with cardiac disease. In Kinney MR and others: *Comprehensive cardiac care,* St Louis, 1991, Mosby–Year Book.

204. Glover J: *Human sexuality in nursing care,* New York, 1985, Appleton-Century-Crofts.

205. Goldenberg I, Goldenberg H: *Family therapy: an overview,* ed 3, Pacific Grove, Calif, 1991, Brooks/Cole.

206. Googe MD, Hinkley CM: Nursing management of adults experiencing musculoskeletal trauma and surgery. In Burrell LO, ed: *Adult nursing in hospital and community settings,* Norwalk, Conn, 1992, Appleton & Lange.

207. Gordon M: Assessing activity tolerance, *Am J Nurs* 76(1):72, 1976.

208. Gordon RE, Gordon KK: Assessing the elements of biopsychosocial functioning, *Hosp Community Psychiatry* 42(5):508, 1991.

209. Gordon VC, Ledray LE: Growth support-intervention for the treatment of depression in women of middle years, *West J Nurs Res* 8(3):263, 1986.

210. Gosnell D: Assessment and evaluation of pressure sores, *Nurs Clin North Am* 22(2):399, June 1987.

211. Govani LE, Hayes JE: *Drugs and nursing implications,* ed 5, Norwalk, Conn, 1988, Appleton-Century-Crofts.

212. Grainger RD: Conquering fears and phobias, *Am J Nurs* 91(5):15, 1991.

213. Grandjean E: Fatigue—its physiological and psychological significance, *Ergonomics* 11(5):427, 1988.

214. Graves L: Diabetic ketoacidosis and hyperosmolar hyperglycemic nonketotic coma, *Crit Care Nurse Q* 13(3):50, 1990.

215. Gray M: Reflex incontinence. In Thompson JM, McFarland GK, Hirsch JE, and others: *Mosby's clinical nursing reference,* ed 2, St Louis, 1989, Mosby–Year Book.

215a. Gray M: Stress incontinence. In Thompson JM, McFarland GK, Hirsch JE, and others: *Mosby's clinical nursing reference,* ed 2, St Louis, 1989, Mosby–Year Book.

216. Gray M: Total incontinence. In Thompson JM, McFarland GK, Hirsch JE, and others: *Mosby's clinical nursing reference,* ed 2, St Louis, 1989, Mosby–Year Book.

217. Greater Milwaukee Area Chapter of AACN, Members of research committee: Fluid volume deficit: validating the indicators, 19(2):152, 1990.

218. Griffin J: Nursing care of the critically ill immunocompromised patient, *Crit Care Q* 9(1):25, 1986.

219. Griffith JL, Griffith ME: Structural family therapy in chronic illness, *Psychosomatics* 28:202, 1987.

220. Groer M: Psychoneuroimmunology, *Am J Nurs* 91(8):33, 1991.

221. Groer M, Shekleton M: *Basic pathophysiology: a holistic approach,* ed 3, St Louis, 1989, Mosby–Year Book.

222. Gulanick M, Ruback C: Shock management. In Bulechek GM, McCloskey JC, eds: *Nursing interventions essential nursing treatments,* ed 2, Philadelphia, 1992, WB Saunders.

223. Gurevich I, Tafuro P: Nursing measures for the prevention of infection in the compromised host, *Nurs Clin North Am* 20(1):257, 1985.

224. Hackett TP, Cassem NH, Wishnic HA: The coronary care unit—an appraisal of its psychologic hazards, *N Engl J Med* 279:1365, 1968.

225. Hahn K: Sexuality and COPD, *Rehabil Nurs* 14(4):191, 1989.

226. Hall J, Weaver B, eds: *Nursing of families in crisis,* Philadelphia, 1974, JB Lippincott.

227. Halpern LM: Analgesic and anti-inflammatory medications. In Tollison CD, ed: *Handbook of chronic pain management,* Baltimore, 1989, Williams & Wilkins.

228. Halpern R: Poverty and early childhood parenting: toward a framework for intervention, *Amer J Orthopsychiatr* 60:6, 1990.

229. Hammond W: Infections in the compromised host, *Hosp Med* 19(10):132, 1983.

230. Hampe S: Needs of the grieving spouse in a hospital setting, *Nurs Res* 24:113, 1975.

231. Hanley MV, Rudd T, Butler J: What happens to intratracheal saline instillations? *Am Rev Respir Dis* 117(2):124, 1978.

232. Hanley MV, Tyler ML: Ineffective airway clearance related to airway infection, *Nurs Clin North Am* 22(1):135, 1987.

233. Harborview Anger Management Program: Helping angry and violent people manage their emotions and behavior, *Hosp Community Psychiatry* 38:1207, 1987.

234. Hardy JB, Streett R: Family support and parenting education in the home: an effective extension of clinic-based preventive health care services for poor children, *J Pediatr* 115:927, 1989.

235. Hartfield MT, Cason CL, Cason GJ: Effect of information about a threatening procedure on patients' expectations and emotional distress, *Nurs Res* 31(4):202, 1982.

236. Haylock RJ, Hart LK: Fatigue in patients receiving localized radiation, *Cancer Nurse* 2(6):461, 1979.

237. Hayter-Muncy J: Measures to rid sleeplessness, *J Gerontol Nurs* 12:6, 1986.

238. Heffline M: A comparative study of pharmacological versus nursing interventions in the treatment of postanesthesia shivering, *J Post Anesthes Nurs* 6(5):311, 1991.

239. Heinicke CM: Toward generic principles of treating patients and children: integrating psychotherapy with the school-aged child and early family intervention, *J Consult Clin Psychol* 58(6):713, 1990.

240. Heldt G: The effect of gavage feeding on the mechanics of the lung, chest wall, and diaphragm of preterm infants, *Pediatr Res* 24:55, 1988.

241. Hennessy K: HHNK dehydration, *Am J Nurs* 83(10):1425, 1983.

242. Herman JA: Nursing assessment and nursing diagnosis in patients with peripheral vascular disease, *Nurs Clin North Am* 21(2):219, 1986.

243. Hernandez M, Miller J: How to reduce falls, *Geriatr Nurs* 7(2):97, 1986.

244. Herth K: Relationship of hope, coping styles, concurrent losses, and setting to grief resolution in the elderly widow(er), *Res Nurs Health* 13:109, 1990.

376

245. Hess L: Nutritional care of the geriatric patient, *J Home Health Care Pract* 2(1):29, 1989.

246. Hilt NE and others: Nursing management of adults with common problems of musculoskeletal system. In Burrell LO, ed: *Adult nursing in hospital and community settings,* Norwalk, Conn, 1992, Appleton & Lange.

247. Hoff LA: *People in crisis: understanding and helping,* Toronto, 1978, Addison-Wesley.

248. Hoffman AL: Diversional activity deficit. In McFarland GK, Thomas MD, eds: *Psychiatric mental health nursing: application of the nursing process,* Philadelphia, 1991, JB Lippincott.

249. Hoffman LA and others: Transtracheal delivery of oxygen: efficacy and safety for long-term continuous therapy, *Ann Otol Rhinol Larynlgol* 100(2):108, 1991.

250. Hogan RM: *Human sexuality. A nursing perspective,* New York, 1985, Appleton-Century-Crofts.

251. Holloway GA and others: Multicenter trial of cadexomer iodine to treat venous stasis ulcer, *West J Med* 151(1):35, 1989.

252. Holmes R and others: Combatting pressure sores—nutritionally, 87(10):1301, 1987.

253. Holtzclaw B: Shivering, *Nurs Clin North Am* 25(4):977, 1990.

254. Hood LE: Interferon. Getting in the way of viruses and tumors, *Am J Nurs* 87(4):459, 1987.

255. Horner J and others: Aspiration following stroke: clinical correlates and outcome, *Neurology* 38(9):1359, 1988.

256. Hoskins LM and others: Mobility, impaired physical. In Thompson JM, McFarland GK, Hirsch JE, and others: *Clinical nursing,* St Louis, 1986, Mosby–Year Book.

257. Hotter A: Wound healing and immunocompromise, *Nurs Clin North Am* 25(1):193, 1990.

258. Hough D, Crosat S, Nye P: Patient education for total hip replacement, *Nurs Manage* 22(3):80I-J, N, P, 1991.

259. Howard M, Puri V, Paidipaty B: The effects of fluid resuscitation in the critically ill patient, *Heart Lung* 13(6):649, 1984.

260. Howie J: How and when should I respond to postop fever? *Am J Nurs* 89(7):984, 1989.

261. Hrobsky DM: Transition to parenthood: a balancing of needs, *Nurs Clin North Am* 12:457, 1977.

262. Humenick SS: The clinical significance of breastmilk maturation rates, *Birth* 14:174, 1987.

263. Humenick SS, Bugen LA: Parenting roles: expectation versus reality, *MCN* 12:36, 1987.

264. Huston CJ: Action stat-hypothermia, *Nursing* 20(12):33, 1990.

265. Hymonovich DP: The chronicity impact and coping instrument: parent questionnaire for use by clinicians and researchers, *Nurs Res* 32:275, 1983.

266. Ignatavicius D, Bayne M: *Medical-surgical nursing: a nursing process approach,* Philadelphia, 1991, WB Saunders.

267. Innes EM: Maintaining fall prevention, *QRB* 11(7):217, 1988.

268. Jack LW: Using play in psychiatric rehabilitation, *J Psychosoc Nurs* 25(7):17, 1987.

269. Jacox A, ed: *Pain: a source book for nurses and other health professionals,* Boston, 1977, Little, Brown & Co.

270. Jaffe M: Geriatric nursing care plans, El Paso, Tex, 1991, Skidmore-Roth Publishing.

271. Jakob DF: Nursing diagnosis case study: community system as client. In Hurley ME, ed: *Classification of nursing diagnoses: proceedings of sixth conference,* St Louis, 1986, Mosby–Year Book.

272. Janelli LM: The impact of health status on body image in older women, *Rehabil Nurs* 13:178, 1988.

273. Janis H, Mann I: *Decision making,* New York, 1977, The Free Press.

274. Janken JI, Reynolds BA: Identifying patients with the potential for falling. In McLane AM, ed: *Classification of nursing diagnoses: proceedings of the seventh conference,* St Louis, 1987, Mosby–Year Book.

275. Janosik EH, Davies JL: *Psychiatric mental health nursing,* Boston, 1989, Jones & Barlett.

276. Janssen JA, Giberson DL: Remotivation therapy, *J Gerontol Nurs* 14(6):31, 1988.

277. Jenny J, Logan J: Analyzing expert nursing practice to develop a new nursing diagnosis: dysfunctional ventilatory weaning response. In Carroll-Johnson RM, ed: *Classification of nursing diagnoses: proceedings of the ninth conference,* Philadelphia, 1991, JB Lippincott.

278. Johnson JL, Morse JM: Regaining control: the process of adjustment after myocardial infarction, *Heart Lung* 19(2):126, 1990.

279. Johnston JF: The elderly and fall prevention, *Appl Nurs Res* 1(3):140, 1987.

280. Junginger J: Predicting compliance with command hallucinations, *Am J Psychiatry* 147(2):245, 1990.

281. Kalbach LR: Unilateral neglect: mechanisms and nursing care, *J Neuroscience Nurs* 23:125, 1991.

282. Kanas N: Therapy group for schizophrenics. In Wells RA, Giannetti UJ, eds: *Handbook of the brief psychotherapies,* New York, 1990, Plenum Press.

283. Kaplan IH, Sadock BJ: *Comprehensive textbook of psychiatry/V,* vol 1, ed 5, Baltimore, 1989, Williams & Wilkins.

284. Kavanaugh KL and others: *Post-discharge experience of breastfeeding a preterm infant.* (Unpublished data).

285. Keckeisen ME, Nyamathi AM: Coping and adjustment to illness in the acute myocardial infarction patient, *J Cardiovasc Nurs* 5(1):25, 1990.

286. Keenan CC: Loss of mobility. In Infante MS, ed: *Crisis theory: a framework for nursing practice,* Reston, Va, 1982, Reston.

287. Keeney RL: Decision analysis: an overview, *Operations Res* 30:803, 1982.

287a. Kersten L: Changes in self-concept during pulmonary rehabilitation, Part I, *Heart Lung* 19(5):456, 1990.

288. Kersten L: Changes in self-concept during pulmonary rehabilitation, Part II, *Heart Lung* 19(5):463, 1990.

289. Kikta MJ and others: A prospective, randomized trial of Unna's boots versus hydroactive dressing in the treatment of venous stasis ulcers, *J Vasc Surg* 7(3):478, 1988.

290. Killian KJ, Jones NL: Respiratory muscles and dyspnea, *Clin Chest Med* 9:237, 1988.

291. Kim MJ, McFarland GK, McLane AM: Pocket guide to nursing diagnoses, ed 4, St Louis, 1991, Mosby–Year Book.

378

292. Kinney AB, Blount M: Effect of cranberry juice on urinary pH, *Nurs Res* 28:287, 1979.

293. Kinney AB, Blount M, Dowell M: Urethral catheterization: pros and cons of an invasive but sometimes essential procedure, *Geriatr Nurs* 1:258, 1980.

294. Kinney CK, Mannettu R, Carpenter MA: Support groups. In Bulechek GM, McCloskey JC, eds: *Nursing interventions: essential nursing treatments,* ed 2, Philadelphia, 1992, WB Saunders.

295. Kinzie JD: The psychiatric effects of massive trauma on Cambodian refugees. In Wilson JP, Harel Z, Kahana B, eds: *Human adaptation to extreme stress,* New York, 1988, Plenum Publishing.

296. Kinzie JD: Therapeutic approaches to traumatized Cambodian refugees, *J Traum Stress* 2(1):75, 1989.

297. Kirilloff LH and others: Does chest physical therapy work? *Chest* 88:436, 1985.

298. Knafl KA, Cavallari KA, Dixon DM: *Pediatric hospitalization: family and nurse perspectives,* Glenview, Ill, 1988, Scott Foresman.

299. Knafl KA, Deatrick JA: Family management style: concept analysis and development, *J Pediatr Nurs* 5:4, 1990.

300. Knebel AR: Weaning from mechanical ventilation: current controversies, *Heart Lung* 20(4):321, 1991.

301. Kobashi-Schoot JAM and others: Assessment of malaise in cancer patients treated with chemotherapy, *Cancer Nurs* 8(6):3, 1985.

302. Konig P: Spacer devices used with metered-dose inhalers breakthrough or gimmick? *Chest* 88:276, 1985.

303. Konstantinides NN, Shronts E: Managing the basics, *Am J Nurs* 1313, 1983.

304. Koontz E, Cox D, Hastings S: Implementing a short-term family support group, *J Psychosoc Nurs Ment Health Serv* 29(5):5, 1991.

305. Krupp LB and others: A study of fatigue in SLE, *J Rheumatol* 17(11):1450, 1990.

306. Kunnel M and others: Comparisons of rectal, femoral, axillary and skin-to-mattress temperatures in stable neonates, *Nurs Res* 37(3):162, 1988.

307. Ladewig PW, London ML, Olds SB: *Essentials of maternal-newborn nursing,* ed 2, Redwood City, Calif, 1990, Addison-Wesley.

308. Lambert C, Lambert V: Psychosocial impacts created by chronic illness, *Nurs Clin North Am* 22(3):527, 1987.

309. Lambert V, Lambert C: *Psychosocial care of the physically ill: what every nurse should know,* ed 2, Englewood Cliffs, NJ, 1985, Prentice-Hall.

310. Lameier DM: Sex and the patient with cardiovascular disease. In Baas LS: *Essentials of cardiovascular nursing,* Gaithersburg, Md, 1991, Aspen Publishers.

311. Lanza ML: Factors relevant to patient assault, *Issues Ment Health Nurs* 9:239, 1988.

312. Lanza M: Origins of aggression, *J Psychosoc Nurs Ment Health Serv* 21:11, 1983.

313. Lapinski ML: Cardiovascular drugs and the elderly population, *Heart Lung* 11(5):430, 1982.

314. Larkin J: Factors influencing one's ability to adapt to chronic illness, *Nurs Clin North Am* 22(3):543, 1987.

315. Larson JL and others: Inspiratory muscle training with a pressure threshold breathing device in patients with chronic obstructive pulmonary disease, *Am Rev Respir Dis* 138:689, 1988.

316. Lawrence RA: *Breastfeeding: a guide for the medical profession,* ed 3, St Louis, 1989, Mosby–Year Book.

317. Lazare A: Bereavement and unresolved grief. In Lazare A, ed: *Outpatient psychiatry: diagnosis and treatment,* ed 2, Baltimore, 1989, Williams & Wilkins.

318. Lazarus RS: The costs and benefits of denial. In Breznitz S, ed: *The denial of stress,* New York, 1983, International Universities Press.

319. Lazarus RS, Folkman S: *Stress, appraisal and coping,* New York, 1986, Springer Publishing.

319a. Lean GR, Chamberlain K: Comparison of daily eating habits and emotional status of overweight persons successful or unsuccessful in maintaining a weight loss, *J Consult Clin Psychol* 61:108, 1973.

320. Ledray LE: A nursing developed model for the treatment of rape victims. In From accommodation to self-determination: nursing's role in the development of health care policy, Kansas City, Mo, 1982, American Academy of Nursing.

321. Ledray LE: Counseling rape victims: the nursing challenge, *Perspec Psychiatric Care* 26(2):21, 1990.

322. Lee E: Cultural factors in working with Southeast Asian refugee adolescents, *J Adolesc* 11(2):167, 1988.

323. Lego S, ed: *The American handbook of psychiatric nursing,* Philadelphia, 1984, JB Lippincott.

324. Leininger M: Becoming aware of types of health practitioners and cultural imposition, *J Transcult Nurs* 2(2):32, 1991.

325. LeMone P: Analysis of a human phenomenon: self-concept, *Nurs Diagnosis* 2(3):126, 1991.

326. Lentz M: Selected aspects of deconditioning secondary to immobilization, *Nurs Clin North Am* 16(4):729, 1981.

327. Leske JS: Hyperglycemic hyperosmolar nonketototic coma: a nursing care plan, *Crit Care Nurse* 5(5):49, 1985.

328. L'Esperance C, Frantz K: Time limitation for early breastfeeding, *JOGNN* 14(2):114, 1985.

329. Liberman RP, DeRisi WJ, Mueser KT: *Social skills training for psychiatric patients,* New York, 1989, Pergamon Press.

330. Liberman RP, Phipps CC: Innovative treatment and rehabilitation techniques for the chronically mentally ill. In Menninger WN, Hannah CT: *The chronic mentally ill,* Washington, DC, 1987, American Psychiatric Press.

331. Lichstein KL, Johnson RS: Older adults' objective self-reporting of sleep in the home, *Behav Ther* 22:531, 1991.

332. Lindgren CL: Burnout and social support in family caregivers, *West J Nurs Res* 12(4):469, 1990.

333. Lion EM: *Human sexuality in nursing process,* New York, 1985, John Wiley & Sons.

334. Lipman TH: Assessing family strengths to guide plan of care using Hymovich's framework, *J Pediatr Nurs* 4:186, 1989.

335. Logan J, Jenny J: Deriving a new nursing diagnosis through qualitative research: dysfunctional ventilatory weaning response, *Nurs Diagnosis* 1(1):37, 1990.

336. Logan J, Jenny J: Interventions for the nursing diagnosis dysfunctional ventilatory weaning response. In Carroll-Johnson RM, ed: *Classification of nursing diagnoses: proceedings of the ninth conference,* Philadelphia, 1991, JB Lippincott.

337. Logemann J and others: The benefit of head rotation on pharyngoesophageal dysphagia, *Arch Phys Med Rehabil* 70:767, 1989.

338. Lohmann M: Fever: different types, different causes, *Nursing* 18(4):98, 1988.

339. Lubkin IM: *Chronic illness: impact and intervention,* Boston, 1991, Jones & Bartlett.

340. Luce J, Tyler M, Pierson D: Therapy to improve airway clearance. In Luce J, Tyler M, Pierson D, eds: *Intensive respiratory care,* Philadelphia, 1984, WB Saunders.

341. Luckmann J, Sorensen K: *Medical-surgical nursing,* ed 3, Philadelphia, 1987, WB Saunders.

342. Lumley W: Controlling hypoglycemia and hyperglycemia, *Nursing* 18(10):34, 1988.

343. Lysaght R, Bodenhamer E: The use of relaxation training to enhance functional outcomes in adults with traumatic head injuries, *Am J Occup Ther* 44(9):797, 1990.

344. Maas M, Specht J: Bowel incontinence. In Maas M, Buckwalter KC, Hardy M, eds: *Nursing diagnosis and interventions for the elderly,* Redwood City, Calif, 1991, Addison-Wesley.

345. Mador MJ, Acevedo FA: Effect of respiratory muscle fatigue on breathing pattern during incremental exercise, *Am Rev Respir Dis* 143:462, 1991.

346. Maier G and others: A model for understanding and managing cycles of aggression among psychiatric patients, *Hosp Community Psychiatry* 38:520, 1987.

347. Maklebust J: Pressure ulcer update, *RN* 54(12):56, 1991.

348. Maklebust J: Pressure ulcers: etiology and prevention, *Nurs Clin North Am* 22(2):359, 1987.

349. Mandelstam D: Special techniques: strengthening pelvic floor muscles, *Geriatr Nurs* 1:251, 1980.

350. Manderino M, Bzdek V: Social skill building with chronic patients, *J Psychosoc Nurs Ment Health Serv* 25(9):18, 1987.

351. Marini JJ: The physiologic determinants of ventilator dependency, *Respir Care* 31:271, 1986.

352. Marini J: *Respiratory medicine for the house officer,* ed 2, Baltimore, 1987, Williams & Wilkins.

353. Marini JJ and others: Weaning from mechanical ventilation. *Am Rev Respir Disease* 138:1043, 1988.

354. Marini J and others: Influence of head dependent positions on lung volume and oxygen saturation in chronic airflow obstruction, *Am Rev Respir Dis* 129:101, 1984.

355. Maslow A: *Motivation and personality,* New York, 1954, Harper & Brothers.

356. Masterson J: *Psychotherapy of the borderline adult,* New York, 1976, Brunner/Mazel.

357. Mayberry JC and others: Fifteen-year results of ambulatory compression therapy for chronic venous ulcers, *Surgery* 100(5):575, 1991.

358. McArthur MJ: Reality therapy with rape victims, *Arch Psychiatr Nurs* 6:360, 1990.

359. McCaffery M: *Nursing management of the patient with pain,* ed 2, Philadelphia, 1979, JB Lippincott.

360. McCann ME: Sexual healing after heart attack, *Am J Nurs* 89(9):1133, 1989.

361. McClave S and others: Use of residual volume as a marker for enteral feeding intolerance: prospective blinded comparison with physical examination and radiographic findings, *Journal Parenter Enter Nutr* 16(2):99, 1992.

362. McCormick K, Burgio KL: Incontinence: update on nursing care measures, *J Gerontol Nurs* 10:16, 1984.

363. McCormick KA, Scheve AAS, Leahy E: Nursing management of urinary incontinence in geriatric patients, *Nurs Clin North Am* 23(1):231, 1988.

364. McCourt AE: The measurement of functional deficit in quality assurance, *Quality Assurance Update* 5(3):1, 1981.

365. McCoy R and others: Nursing management of breast feeding for preterm infants, *J Perinat Neonat Nurs* 2:42, 1988.

366. McCubbin H, Patterson J, eds: *Systematic assessment of family stress: resources and coping,* St Paul, 1981, University of Minnesota.

367. McCullough FL, Evans LM: Assessment of neurovascular status in children, *Orthop Nurs* 4(4):19, 1985.

368. McElroy A, Townsend PK: Health repercussions of culture contact. In *Medical anthropology in ecological perspective,* ed 2, Boulder, Colo, 1989, Westview Press.

369. McFarland GK, Naschinski C: Impaired communication: a descriptive study, *Nurs Clin North Amer* 20(4):775, 1985.

370. McFarland GK, Naschinski C: Communication. In Thompson JM, McFarland GK, Hirsch JE, and others: *Clinical nursing,* ed 3, St Louis, 1992, Mosby–Year Book.

371. McFarland GK, Wasli EL, Gerety EK: *Nursing diagnoses and process in psychiatric mental health nursing,* Philadelphia, 1992, JB Lippincott.

372. McGuire TJ, Kramer VN: Autonomic dysreflexia in the spinal cord injured: what every physician should know about this medical emergency, *Postgrad Med* 80(2):81, 1986.

373. McInnis M, Marks I: Audiotape therapy for persistent auditory hallucinations, *Br J Psychiatry* 157:913, 1990.

374. McIntosh WA, Shifflett PA, Pecore JS: Social support, stressful events, strain, dietary intake, and the elderly, *Medical Care* 27(2):140, 1989.

375. McLane AM, McShane RE: Empirical validation of defining characteristics of constipation: a study of bowel elimination practices of healthy adults. In Hurley M, ed: *Classification of nursing diagnoses: proceedings of the sixth conference,* St Louis, 1986, Mosby–Year Book.

376. McLane AM, McShane RE: Constipation. In Maas M, Buckwalter KC, Hardy M, eds: *Nursing diagnosis and intervention for the elderly,* Redwood City, Calif, 1991, Addison-Wesley.

377. McLane AM, McShane RE: Elimination. In Thompson JM, McFarland GK, Hirsch JE, and others: *Clinical nursing,* ed 2, St Louis, 1989, Mosby–Year Book.

378. McLane AM, McShane RE: Bowel management. In Bulechek GM, McCloskey JC, eds: *Nursing interventions: essential nursing treatments,* Philadelphia, 1992, WB Saunders.

379. McShane RE, McLane AM: Constipation: impact of etiological factors, *J Gerontol Nurs* 14(4):31, 1988.

380. McShane RE, McLane AM: Constipation: consensual and empirical validation, *Nurs Clin North Am* 20:80, 1985.

381. Meier PP: Bottle and breast feeding: effects on transcutaneous oxygen pressure and temperature in preterm infants, *Nurs Res* 37:36, 1988.

382. Meier PP, Brennan-Behm M: *Management of enteral feeding for preterm infants: a literature review.* (Manuscript submitted for publication).

383. Meier PP, Mangurten HH: Management of breastfeeding for "special care" infants. In Riordan J, Auerbach KS, eds: *Breast feeding and human milk,* Jones & Bartlett (in press).

384. Meier PP, Pugh EJ: Breast feeding behavior of small preterm infants, *MCN* 10:396, 1985.

385. Meier PP, Wilks SO: The bacteria in expressed mothers milk, *MCN* 12:420, 1987.

386. Meier PP and others: Bottle and breastfeeding: physiologic effects on preterm infants (abstract), *Neonatal Network* 10:78, 1991.

387. Meier PP and others: *A model to support breast feeding in neonatal intensive care.* (Manuscript submitted for publication).

388. Meinhart NT, McCaffery M: *Pain: a nursing approach to assessment and analysis,* Norwalk, Conn, 1983, Appleton-Century-Crofts.

389. Menaghan EG: Individual coping efforts and family studies: conceptual and methodological issues. In McCubbin HI, Sussman MB, Patterson JM, eds: *Social stress and the family: advances and developments in family stress theory and research,* New York, 1983, The Haworth Press.

390. Merenstein G, Gardner S: *Handbook of neonatal intensive care,* St Louis, 1985, Mosby–Year Book.

391. Merskey H: Development of a universal language of pain syndromes. In Bonica JJ and others, eds: *Advances in pain research and therapy,* vol 5, New York, 1978, Raven Press.

392. Metheny NA, Eisenberg P, Spies M: Aspiration pneumonia in patients fed through nasoenteral tubes, *Heart Lung* 15(3):256, 1986.

393. Meyers K, Hickey MK: Nursing management of hypovolemic shock, *Crit Care Nurse Q* 11(1):57, 1988.

394. Michael Reese Hospital and Medical Center: Nursing care plans: nursing diagnosis and intervention. In Gulanick M, Klopp A, Galanes S, eds: St Louis, 1986, Mosby–Year Book.

395. Mickus P: Activities of daily living in women after myocardial infarction, *Heart Lung* 15:376, 1986.

396. Miller B, Evans W: Nurse and patient: allies in preventing amputation, *RN* 51(7):38, 1988.

397. Miller F and others: A preliminary study of unresolved grief in families of seriously mentally ill patients, *Hosp Community Psychiatry* 41(12):1321, 1990.

398. Miller JF: *Coping with chronic illness: overcoming powerlessness,* ed 2, Philadelphia, 1991, FA Davis.

399. Miller NH: Cardiac rehabilitation. In Kinney MR and others: *Comprehensive cardiac care,* St Louis, 1991, Mosby–Year Book.

400. Miller P and others: Influence of a nursing intervention on regimen adherence and societal adjustment post myocardial infarction, *Nurs Res* 37(5):297, 1988.

401. Mills PD, Hansen JC: Short-term group interventions for mentally ill young adults living in a community residence and their families, *Hosp Community Psychiatry,* 42(11):1144, 1991.

402. Mitchell M: Neuroscience nursing—a nursing diagnosis approach, Baltimore, 1989, Williams & Wilkins.

403. Moon JL, Humenick SS: Breast engorgement: contributing variables and variables amenable to nursing intervention, *J Obstet Gynecol Neonat Nurs* 18(4):309, 1989.

404. Morgan SP: A comparison of three methods of managing fever in the neurologic patient, *J Neurosci Nurs* 22(1):19, 1990.

405. Morin CM, Kowatch RA, O'Shanick G: Sleep restriction for the inpatient treatment of insomnia, *Sleep* 13(2):183, 1990.

406. Morrison EF: Theoretical modeling to predict violence in hospitalized psychiatric patients, *Res Nurs Health* 12:31-40, 1989.

407. Morse JM, Harrison MJ: Social coercion for weaning, *J Nurse Midwife* 32(4):205, 1987.

408. Moss RC: Overcoming fear—a review of research on patient, family instruction, *AORN J* 43(5):1107, 1986.

409. Mourad LA, Droste MM: *The nursing process in the care of adults with orthopaedic conditions,* New York, 1988, John Wiley & Sons.

410. Mueller RE, Petty TL, Filley GF: Ventilation and arterial blood gas changes induced by pursed lips breathing, *J Appl Physiol* 28:784, 1970.

411. Mullan H, Roubenoff RA, Roubenoff R: Risks of pulmonary aspiration among patients receiving enteral nutrition support, *J Parenter Enter Nutri* 16(2):160, 1992.

412. Munro B and others: Effect of relaxation therapy on post-myocardial infarction patients' rehabilitation, *Nurs Res* 37:4, 1988.

413. Murray RB, Huelskoetter MMW: *Psychiatric—mental health nursing,* Connecticut, 1897, Appleton & Lange.

414. Murray S, Thompson R: We've organized our approach to pressure sores, *RN* 54(1):42, 1991.

415. Nagai-Jacobsen MG, Burkhardt MA: Spirituality: cornerstone of holistic nursing practice, *Holistic Nurs Prac* 3(3):18, 1989.

416. Nail LM, King KB: Fatigue, *Semin Oncol Nurs* 3(4):257-262.

417. Naschinski C: Hopelessness. In Thompson JM and others: *Mosby's manual of clinical nursing,* ed 3, St Louis, 1992, Mosby–Year Book.

418. Naschinski C, McFarland GK: Impaired verbal communication. In McFarland GK, McFarlane EA: *Nursing diagnosis and intervention: planning for patient care,* ed 2, St Louis, 1992, Mosby–Year Book.

419. Neifert M, Seacat J: Contemporary breast-feeding management, *Clin Perinatol* 12(2):319, 1985.

420. Neifert MA, Seacat J: *Milk yield and prolactin rise with simultaneous breast pump,* Abstracted from the Ambulatory Pediatric Association Annual Meeting, Washington, DC, May 7-10, 1985.

421. Neill KM: The need for safety. In Yura H, Walsh MB, eds: *Human needs 3 and the nursing process,* Norwalk, Conn, 1983, Appleton-Century-Crofts.

422. Nelson HE, Thrasher S, Barnes TR: Practical ways of alleviating auditory hallucinations, *BMJ* 302(6772):327, 1991.

423. Nelson PB: Ethnic differences in intrinsic/extrinsic religious orientation and depression in the elderly, *Arch Psychiatr Nurs* 3(4):199, 1989.

384

424. Newell B: Body-image disturbance: cognitive behavioural formulation and intervention, *J Adv Nurs* 16:1400, 1991.

425. Newton M, Newton N: Postpartum engorgement of the breast, *Am J Obstet Gynecol* 61(3):664, 1951.

426. Nickens H: Intrinsic factors in falling among the elderly, *Arch Intern Med* 145:1089, 1985.

427. Nocturnal oxygen therapy trial group: Continuous or nocturnal oxygen therapy in hypoxemic chronic obstructive lung disease: a clinical trial, *Ann Intern Med* 93:391, 1980.

428. Nolde T, Wong S, Wong J: Teaching patients to use a new hip, *Geriatr Nurs,* 69, March/April 1989.

429. Norris J, Kunes-Connell M: Self-esteem disturbance, *Nurs Clin North Am* 20(4):745, 1985.

430. Norris J, Kunes-Connell M: A multimodal approval, validation and refinement of an existing nursing diagnosis, *Arch Psychiatr Nurs* 2(2):103, 1988.

431. Northouse LL: Social support in patient's and husband's adjustment to breast cancer, *Nurs Res* 37(2):91, 1988.

432. Northouse LL, Cracchiolo-Caraway A, Pappas Appel C: Psychologic consequences of breast cancer on partner and family, *Semin Oncol Nurs* 7(3):216, 1991.

433. Norton C: Incontinence in the elderly. IV. Nursing the incontinent patient, *Nurs Times Suppl* 81(1):13, 1985.

434. Norton L, Comforti CG: The effects of body position on oxygenation, *Heart Lung* 14:45, 1985.

435. Nuernberger P: *Freedom from stress: a holistic approach,* Honesdale, Pa, 1981, The Himalayan International Institute of Yoga Science and Philosphy.

436. Nyamathi A, Kashiwabara A: Preoperative anxiety—its effect on cognitive thinking, *AORN J* 47(1):164, 1988.

437. O'Donoghue PD: The child and family at psychosocial risk. In Mott SR, James SR, Sperhac AM: *Nursing care of children and families,* ed 2, Redwood City, Calif, 1990, Addison-Wesley.

438. O'Donovan P, O'Brien N: Group B Beta haemolytic disease in preterm twins associated with the ingestion of infected breast milk: a case report, *Ir J Med Sci* 154:158, 1985.

439. Oliver S, Fuessel E: Control of postoperative hypothermia in cardiovascular surgery patients, *Crit Care Nurs Q* 12(4):63, 1990.

440. Olshansky EF: Parenting, altered. In McFarland GK, Thomas MD: *Psychiatric mental health nursing: application of the nursing process,* New York, 1991, JB Lippincott.

441. Olson D and others: *Families: what makes them work,* Beverly Hills, Calif, 1983, Sage.

442. Olson E, ed: The hazards of immobility, *Am J Nurs* 67(4):780, 1967.

443. Omer GE: Assessment of hand trauma, *Orthop Nurs* 4(4):29, 1985.

444. Oncology Nursing Society, American Nurses Association: *Outcome standards for cancer nursing practice,* Kansas City, Mo, 1987, The Association.

445. Orr P: An educational program for total hip and knee replacement patients as part of a total arthritis center program, *Orthop Nurs* 9(5):61, 1990.

446. Paloutzian R, Ellison C: Loneliness, spiritual well-being, and quality of life. In Peplau L, Perlman D, eds: *Loneliness: a sourcebook of*

current theory, research, and therapy, New York, 1982, John Wiley & Sons.

447. Parkes C: *Bereavement: studies of grief in adult life,* Madison, Conn, 1987, International Universities Press.

448. Peck SA: Crush syndrome: pathophysiology and mangement, *Orthop Nurs* 9(3):33, 1990.

449. Pender NJ: Self-modification. In Bulechek GM, McCloskey J, eds: *Nursing interventions: treatment for nursing diagnoses,* Philadelphia, 1985, WB Saunders.

450. Pender NJ: *Health promotion in nursing practice,* ed 2, Norwalk, Conn, 1987, Appleton-Lange.

451. Pender NJ, Pender AR: Attitudes, subjective norms and intentions to engage in health behaviors, *Nurs Res* 35(1):15, 1986.

452. Pender NJ, Pender AR: Health promotion in nursing practice, ed 2, East Norwalk, Conn, 1987, Appleton & Lange.

453. Peplau H: *Interpersonal relationships in nursing,* New York, 1952, GP Putnam's Sons.

454. Peplau LA, Miceli M, Morasch B: Loneliness and self-evaluation. In Peplau LA, Perlman D, eds: *Loneliness,* New York, 1982, John Wiley & Sons.

455. Peret KK, Stachowiak B: Alteration in health maintenance: conceptual bases, etiology, and defining characteristics. In Kim MJ, McFarland GK, McLane AM, eds: *Classification of nursing diagnoses: proceedings of the fifth national conference,* St Louis, 1984, Mosby–Year Book.

456. Peterson M: Patient anxiety before cardiac catheterization: an intervention study, *Heart Lung* 20(6):643, 1991.

457. Pflaum S: Investigation of intake-output as a means of assessing body fluid balance, *Heart Lung* 8(3):495, 1979.

458. Philichi LM: Family adaptation during a pediatric intensive care hospitalization, *J Pediatr Nurs* 4:268, 1991.

459. Phipps M: Assessment of neurological deficits in stroke, *Nurs Clin North Am* 26(4):957, 1991.

460. Phipps WJ, Long BC, Woods NF: *Medical-surgical nursing: concepts and clinical practice,* St Louis, 1987, Mosby–Year Book.

461. Piccinimo S: The nursing care challenge: borderline patients, *J Psychosoc Nurs* 28(4):22, 1990.

462. Pigg JS, Dricoll PW, Caniff R: *Rheumatology nursing: a problem oriented approach,* New York, 1985, John Wiley & Sons.

463. Pilch J: *Wellness: your invitation to full life,* Minneapolis, 1981, Winston Press.

464. Plante TG: Social skill training: a program to help schizophrenic clients cope, *J Psychosoc Nurs Ment Health Serv* 27(3):6, 1989.

465. Podrasky DL, Sexton DL: Nurses' reactions to difficult patients, *Image J Nurs Sch* 20(1):16, 1988.

466. Pollman JW, Morris JJ, Rose P: Is fiber the answer to constipation problems in the elderly? A review of literature, *Int J Nurs Stud* 15:107, 1978.

467. Pollock GH: The mourning liberation process in health and disease, *Psychiatr Clin North Am* 10(3):345, 1987.

468. Potempa K and others: Chronic fatigue, *Image J Nurs Sch* 18:165, 1986.

386

469. Powers BA: Social networks, social support, and elderly institutionalized people, *Adv in Nurs Sci* 10:40, 1988.

470. Powers MJ, Jalowiec A: Profile of the well-controlled well-adjusted hypertensive patient, *Nurs Res* 36:106, 1987.

471. Poyss AS: Fluid therapy. In Bulechek GM, McCloskey JC, eds: *Nursing interventions: essential nursing treatments,* ed 2, Philadelphia, 1992, WB Saunders.

472. Pradka L: Use of the wick catheter for diagnosing and monitoring compartment syndrome, *Orthop Nurs* 4(4):17, 1985.

473. Preusser RA and others: Effects of two methods of preoxygenation on mean arterial pressure, cardiac output, peak airway pressure, and postsuctioning hypoxemia, *Heart Lung* 17(3):290, 1988.

474. Price B: A model for body-image care, *J Adv Nurs* 15:585, 1990.

475. Prizant-Weston M, Castiglia K: Hemodynamic regulation in nursing interventions. In Bulechek GM, McCloskey JC, eds: *Essential nursing treatments,* Philadelphia, 1992, WB Saunders.

476. Putnam J: Total hip replacement: helping your patient avoid complications, *Nurs Life* 6, March/April 1986.

477. Radebaugh TS, Hadley E, Suzman R, eds: Falls in the elderly: biologic and behavioral aspects, *Clin Geriatr Med* 1:497, 1985.

478. Radtke K: Exercise compliance in cardiac rehabilitation, *Rehabil Nurs* 14:4, 1989.

479. Rakel B: Knowledge deficit. In Maas M, Buckwalter KC, Hardy M, eds: *Nursing diagnoses and interventions for the elderly,* Redwood City, Calif, 1991, Addison-Wesley.

480. Ramey L, Cloud J: Relocation success: a model for mental health counselors, *J Ment Health Couns* 9(3):150, 1987.

481. Rando TA: Anticipatory grief: the term is a misnomer but the phenomenon exists, *J Palliat Care* 4(1,2):70, 1988.

482. Rando TA: *Loss and anticipatory grief,* Lexington, Mass, 1986, Lexington Books.

483. Rathert ML, Talarezyk GJ: Patient compliance with the decision making process of clinicians and patient, *J Compliance Health Care* 2:55, 1987.

484. Ravdin JI, Guerrant RL: Infectious diarrhea in the elderly, *Geriatrics* 38:95, 1983.

485. Redman BK: *The process of patient education,* ed 6, St Louis, 1988, Mosby–Year Book.

486. Reed PG: Mental health of older adults, *West J Nurs Res* 11(2):143, 1989.

487. Reed PG: Spirituality and mental health in older adults: extant knowledge of for nursing, *Fam Community Health* 14(2):14, 1991.

488. Reed-Ash C, Gianella A: Patient education, *Cancer Nurs* 5:261, 1982.

489. Reeder D: Cognitive therapy of anger management: theoretical and practical considerations, *Arch Psychiatr Nurs* 5:147, 1991.

490. Reheis C: Neurtropenia, *Nurs Clin North Am* 20(1):219, 1985.

491. Resnick BM: Geriatric motivation—clinically helping the elderly to comply, *J Gerontol Nurs* 17(5):17, 1991.

492. Rice MA, Szopa TJ: Group intervention for reinforcing self-worth following mastectomy, *Oncol Nurs Forum* 15(1):33, 1988.

493. Richards KC, Brainsfather L: Night sleep patterns in the critical care unit, *Heart Lung* 17(1):35, 1988.

494. Riddoch MJ, Humphreys GW: The effects of cueing on unilateral neglect, *Neuropsychologia* 21(6):589, 1983.

495. Ristuccia A: Hematologic effects of cancer chemotherapy, *Nurs Clin North Am* 20(1):235, 1985.

496. Robertson SM: Self-concept disturbance. In McFarland GK, Thomas MD: *Psychiatric mental health nursing: application of the nursing process,* Philadelphia, 1991, JB Lippincott.

497. Robinson P, Fleming S: Differentiating grief and depression, *Hospice J* 5(1):77, 1989.

498. Rogers CS, Morris S, Taper IJ: Weaning from the breast: influences on maternal decisions, *Pediatric Nurse* 13(5):341, 1987.

499. Rombeau JL, Caldwell MD, eds: *Enteral and tube feeding,* Philadelphia, 1984, WB Saunders.

500. Rombeau JL, Caldwell MD, eds: *Enteral and tube feeding,* ed 2, Philadelphia, 1990, WB Saunders.

501. Romme MAJ, Escher A: Hearing voices, *Schizophrenia Bull* 15(2):209, 1989.

502. Roper M, Anderson N: The interactional dynamics of violence, part I: an acute psychiatric ward, *Arch Psychiatr Nurs* 5:209, 1991.

503. Rosenheim E, Reicher R: Children in anticipatory grief: the lonely predicament, *J Clin Child Psychol* 15(2):115, 1986.

504. Rothert ML, Talarczyk GJ: Patient compliance and the decision making process of clinicians and patients, *J Compliance Health Care* 2:55, 1987.

505. Rousseau E and others: Influence of cultural and environmental factors on breast-feeding, *CMA J* 127:701, 1982.

506. Rubenfeld MG: Diversional activity deficit. In Thompson J, McFarland G, Hirsch J, Tucker S, Bowers A: *Clinical nursing,* ed 2, St Louis, 1989, Mosby–Year Book.

507. Rubenfeld M: Total incontinence. In McFarland GK, McFarlane EA, eds: *Nursing diagnosis and intervention: planning for patient care,* St Louis, 1989, Mosby–Year Book.

508. Rubin JR and others: Unna's vs polyurethane foam dressings for the treatment of venous ulceration. A randomized prospective study, *Arch Surg* 125(4):489, 1990.

509. Ruesch J, Bateson G: *Communication: the social matrix of psychiatry,* New York, 1987, WW Norton.

510. Russel D: The measurement of loneliness. In Peplau LA, Perlman D, eds: *Loneliness,* New York, 1982, John Wiley & Sons.

511. Ryan P: Noncompliance. In Thompson JM, McFarland GK, Hirsch JE, and others: *Clinical nursing,* St Louis, 1986, Mosby–Year Book.

512. Ryan P, Falco S: A pilot study to validate the etiologies and defining characteristics of the nursing diagnosis of noncompliance, *Nurs Clin North Am* 20(4):685, 1985.

513. Sayre J: Psychodynamics revisited: an object-relations framework for psychiatric nursing, *Persp Psychiatr Care* 26(1):7, 1990.

514. Scalzi CC, Burke LE: Sexual counseling. In Underhill SL and others, eds: *Cadiac nursing,* ed 2, Philadelphia, 1989, JB Lippincott.

515. Scandrett-Hibdon S: Cognitive reappraisal. In Bulechek GM, McCloskey JC, eds: *Nursing interventions: essential nursing treatments,* ed 2, Philadelphia, 1992, WB Saunders.

516. Scandrett-Hibdon S, Uecker S: Relaxation training. In Bulechek GM, McCloskey JC, eds: *Nursing interventions: essential nursing treatments,* ed 2, Philadelphia, 1992, WB Saunders.

516a. Schacter SO: Threats of suicide, *J Contemp Psychother* 18(2):145, 1988.

517. Schaefer KM: Care of the patient with congestive heart failure. In Schaefer KM, Benson PJ, eds: Levine's conversation model: a framework for nursing practice, Philadelphia, 1991, FA Davis Co.

518. Scharer KA, Dixon DM: Managing chronic illness: parents with a ventilator-dependent child, *J Pediatr Nurs* 4:236, 1989.

519. Schenk E: Substance abuse. In Phipps WJ, Long BC, Woods NF, eds: *Medical-surgical nursing: concepts and clinical practice,* St Louis, 1987, Mosby–Year Book.

520. Schilder E: Bodily perceptions and their influence on health, *Nurs Standard* 4(13/14):30, 1989.

521. Schroeder P, Gunta K: Comfort, alteration in: pain. In Thompson JM, McFarland GK, Hirsch JE, and others: *Clinical nursing,* St Louis, 1986, Mosby–Year Book.

522. Schwertz DW, Piano MR: New inotropic drugs for treatment of congestive heart failure, *Cardiovasc Nurs* 26(3):7, 1990.

523. Scott J, Williams JMG, Beck AT, eds: *Cognitive therapy in clinical practice: an illustrative casebook,* New York, 1989, Routledge.

524. Sebastian L: Promoting object constancy—writing as a nursing intervention, *J Psychosoc Nurs* 29(1):21, 1991.

524a. Sebree R, Papkess-Vawter S: Self-injury concept formation: nursing diagnosis, *Persp Psychiatr Care* 27(2):27, 1991.

525. Sexton D: *Nursing care of the respiratory patient,* Norwalk, Conn, 1990, Appleton & Lange.

526. Sexton DL, Munro BH: Living with a chronic illness: the experience of women with chronic obstructive pulmonary disease, *West J Nurs Res* 10(1):26, 1988.

527. Sharp JT and others: Thoracoabdominal motion in chronic obstructive pulmonary disease, *Am Rev Respir Dis* 115:47, 1977.

528. Shekleton ME: Respiratory muscle conditioning and the work of breathing: a critical balance in the weaning patient, *AACN Clin Issues Crit Care Nurs* 2(3):405, 1991.

529. Shekleton M: Impaired physical mobility. In Shekleton M, Litwack K, eds: *Critical care nursing of the surgical patient,* Philadelphia, 1991, WB Saunders.

530. Shekleton ME, Nield M: Ineffective airway clearance related to artificial airway, *Nurs Clin North Am* 22(1):167, 1987.

531. Shelp EE, Perl M: Denial in clinical medicine: a reexamination of the concept and its significance, *Arch Intern Med* 145:697, 1985.

532. Shepard AM, Blannin JP, Fineley RCL: Changing attitudes in the management of urinary incontinence: the need for specialist nursing, *Br Med J* 284:645, 1982.

533. Shepard AM, Tribe E, Tarrens MJ: Simple practical techniques in the management of urinary incontinence, *Int Rehabil Med* 4:15, 1982.

534. Sheppard KC: Validation of the diagnosis alterations in protective mechanisms. In Carroll-Johnson R, ed: *Classification of nursing diagnoses: proceedings of the eighth conference,* Philadelphia, 1989, JB Lippincott.

535. Sheppard KC: Alteration in protective mechanisms. In McLane A, ed: *Classification of nursing diagnoses: proceedings of the seventh conference,* St Louis, 1987, Mosby–Year Book.

536. Sheppard KC: Altered protection: a nursing diagnosis. In Carroll-Johnson R, ed: *Classification of nursing diagnoses: proceedings of the ninth conference,* Philadelphia, 1991, JB Lippincott.

537. Sherman DW: Managing an acute head injury, *Nursing,* 20(4):47, 1990.

538. Showers J: Behaviour management cards as a method of anticipatory guidance for parents, *Child Care Health Dev* 15:401, 1989.

539. Shrago L, Bocar D: The infant's contribution to breastfeeding, *J Obstet Gynecol Neonat Nurs* 19(3):209, 1990.

539a. Simon J: The single parent: power and the integrity of parenting, *Am J Psychoanal* 50:187, 1990.

540. Sjogren B, Vdbenberg N: Decision making during the prenatal diagnostic procedure, *Prenat Diagn* 8:263, 1988.

541. Slimmer LW, Brown RT: Parent's decision making process in medication administration for control of hyperactivity, *J School Health* 55:221, 1985.

542. Smith B, Cantrell P: Distance in nurse-patient encounters, *J Psychosoc Nurs Ment Health Serv* 22(2):22, 1988.

543. Smith DAJ: Continence restoration in the homebound patient, *Nurs Clin North Am* 23(1):207, 1988.

544. Gresham S: Clinical assessment and management of swallowing difficulties after stroke, *Med J Aust* 153(7):397, 1990.

545. Sodestrom KE, Martinson IM: Patients' spiritual coping strategies: a study of nurse and patient perspectives, *Oncol Nurs Forum* 14(2):41, 1987.

546. Sommers M: Rapid fluid resuscitation, *Nursing* 20(1):52, 1990.

547. Sparks SM, Taylor CM: *Nursing diagnosis manual: an indispensable guide to better patient care,* Springhouse, Penn, 1991, Springhouse.

548. Speake DL, Cowart ME, Pellet K: Health perceptions and lifestyles of the elderly, *Res Nurs Health* 12:93, 1989.

549. Specht J and others: Urinary incontinence. In Maas M, Buckwalter KC, Hardy M, eds: *Nursing diagnoses and interventions for the elderly,* Redwood City, Calif, 1991, Addison-Wesley.

550. Spencer T and others: *Clinical pharmacology and nursing management,* Philadelphia, 1989, JB Lippincott.

551. Squires R and others: Cardiovascular rehabilitation: status, 1990. *Mayo Clin Proc* 65:731, 1990.

552. Stafford MJ: Monitoring patients with permanent cardiac pacemakers, *Nurs Clin North Am* 22:503, 1987.

553. Standards and guidelines for cardiopulmonary resuscitation and emergency cardiac care, *JAMA* 255(21):2841, 1986.

554. Stanwyck DJ: Self-esteem through the life span, *Fam Community Health* 6(2):11, 1983.

555. Starker JE: Psychosocial aspects of geographic relocation: the development of a new social network, *Am J Health Promot* 5(1):52, 1990.

556. Stechel SB: *Patient contracting,* Norwalk, Conn, 1982, Appleton-Century-Crofts.

557. Steele L: The death surround: factors influencing the grief experience of survivors, *Oncol Nurs Forum* 17(2):235, 1990.

558. Stein RE, Jessop DJ: Long term mental health effects of a pediatric home care program, *Pediatrics* 88:490, 1991.

559. Stewart M: Measurement of clinical pain. In Jacox A, ed: *Pain: a source book for nurses and other health professionals,* Boston, 1977, Little, Brown & Co.

560. Stewart T, Shields CR: Grief in chronic illness: assessment and management, *Arch Phys Med Rehabil* 66:447, 1985.

561. Stiles MK: The shining stranger: nurse-family spiritual relationship, *Cancer Nurs* 13(4):235, 1990.

562. Stinemetz J and others: *Rx for stress: a nurses' guide,* Palo Alto, Calif, 1984, Bull Publishing.

563. Stoner M: Measuring hope. In Stromberg S: *Instruments for clinical nursing practice,* Norwalk, Conn, 1989, Appleton & Lange.

564. Strauss A, Glaser B: *Chronic illness and the quality of life,* St Louis, 1975, Mosby–Year Book.

565. Stuart EM, Deckro JP, Mandle CL: Spirituality in health and healing: a clinical program, *Holistic Nurs Pract* 3(3):35, 1989.

566. Stuifbergen AK: Patterns of functioning in families with a chronically ill parent: an exploratory study, *Res Nurs Health* 13:35, 1990.

567. Swanson J and others: Violence and psychiatric disorder in the community: evidence from the epidemiologic catchment area surveys, *Hosp Community Psychiatry* 41:761, 1990.

568. Swearingen P, ed: *Manual of nursing therapeutics—applying nursing diagnosis to medical disorders,* ed 2, St Louis, 1990, Mosby–Year Book.

569. Sweeting HN, Gilhooly ML: Anticipatory grief: a review, *Soc Sci Med* 30(10):1073, 1990.

570. Tardif GS: Sexual activity after a myocardial infarction, *Arch Phys Med Rehabil* 70(10):763, 1989.

571. Taylor-Loughran AE and others: Defining characteristics of the nursing diagnoses *fear* and *anxiety:* a validation study, *Appl Nurs Res* 2(4):178, 1989.

572. Taylor AG: Pain, *Ann Rev Nurs Res* 5:23, 1987.

573. Teasdale K: The withdrawn schizophrenic, *Nurs Times* 82:32, 1986.

574. Thomas K: The emergence of body temperature biorhythm in preterm infants, *Nurs Res* 40(2):98, 1991.

575. Thomas L: Self-esteem and life satisfaction, *J Gerontol Nurs* 14(12):25, 1988.

576. Thomas SA and others: Denial in coronary care patients—an objective reassessment, *Heart Lung* 12:74, 1983.

577. Thompson M: Injury, potential for. In Thompson JM, McFarland GK, Hirsch JE, and others: *Clinical nursing,* St Louis, 1986, Mosby–Year Book.

578. Thompson JM: Post-trauma response. In Thompson JM, McFarland GK, Hirsch JE, and others: *Clinical nursing,* ed 2, St Louis, 1989, Mosby–Year Book.

579. Thompson JM, McFarland G, Hirsch J, Tucker S, eds: *Mosby's clinical nursing reference,* St Louis, 1987, Mosby–Year Book.

580. Thorpe DM: Sleep disturbances in the cancer patient, *Cancer Bull* 43(5):393, 1991.

581. Tiep BL and others: Pursed lip breathing training using ear oximetry, *Chest* 90:218, 1986.

582. Tischler MD, Smith TW: Digitalis: its current place in the treatment of heart failure, *Mod Concepts Cardiovasc Dis* 59(12):67, 1990.

583. Titler M and others: Classification of nursing interventions for care of the integument, *Nursing Diagnosis* 2(2):45, 1991.

584. Tobin MJ: Weaning from mechanical ventilation. In Simmons DH, ed: *Current pulmonology,* vol 11, St Louis, 1990, Mosby–Year Book.

585. Tobin MJ, Jung K: Weaning from mechanical ventilation, *Crit Care Clin* 6(3):725, 1990.

586. Topf M: Effects of personal control over hospital noise on sleep, *Res Nurs Health* 15(1):19, 1992.

587. Topf M, Dambacher B: Teaching interpersonal skills: a model for facilitating optimal interpersonal relations, *J Psychiatr Nurs Ment Health Serv* 19:29, 1981.

588. Traver GA: Ineffective airway clearance: physiology and clinical application, *Dimens Crit Care Nurs* 4(4):198, 1985.

589. Travis J, Ryan R: *Wellness workbook: a guide to attaining high level wellness,* Berkeley, Calif, 1986, Ten Speed Press.

590. Trelvar DM, Stechmiller J: Pulmonary aspiration in tube-fed patients with artificial airways, *Heart Lung* 13(6):667, 1984.

591. Turner J: Nursing intervention in patients with peripheral vascular disease, *Nurs Clin North Am* 21(2):233, 1986.

592. Turner SL, Plymat KR: As women use: perspectives on urinary incontinence, *Rehabil Nurs* 13(3):132, 1988.

593. Tyler ML: Complications of positioning and chest physiotherapy, *Respir Care* 27:458, 1982.

594. Tyler ML: The respiratory effects of body positioning and immobilization, *Respir Care* 29(5):472, 1984.

595. Twycross RG: Narcotic analgesics in clinical practice. In Bonica JJ and others, eds: *Advances in pain research and therapy,* vol 5, New York, 1983, Raven Press.

595a. Underwood BA: Evaluating the nutritional status of individuals: a critique of approaches, *Nutr Rev Suppl* 213, May 1986.

596. Unger KV and others: A supported education program for young adults with long term mental illness, *Hosp Community Psychiatr* 42(8):838, 1991.

597. van der Schans CP and others: Effect of forced expirations on mucus clearance in patients with chronic airflow obstruction: effect of lung recoil pressure, *Thorax* 45:623, 1990.

598. Van Deusen J: Unilateral neglect, *Am J Occup Ther* 42(7):441, 1988.

599. Varricchio CG: Selecting a tool for measuring fatigue, *Oncol Nurs Forum* 12(4):122, 1985.

600. Voith AM: Alterations in urinary elimination concepts, research and practice, *Rehabil Nurs* 13(3):122, 1988.

601. Voith AM, Smith DA: Validation of the nursing diagnosis of urinary retention, *Nurs Clin North Am* 20:723, 1985.

602. Volden C and others: The relationship of age, gender, and exercise practices to measures of health, life-style, and self-esteem, *Appl Nurs Res* 3(1):20, 1990.

603. Volker D: Neoplasia. In Beare PG, Myers JL, eds: *Principles and practice of adult health nursing,* St Louis, 1990, Mosby–Year Book.

604. Wade B, Bowling A: Appropriate use of drugs by elderly people, *J Adv Nurs* 11:47, 1986.

605. Wadle K: Diarrnea. In Maas M, Buckwalter KC, Hardy M, eds: *Nursing diagnoses and interventions for the elderly,* Redwood City, Calif, 1991, Addison-Wesley.

606. Wake M, Fehring R, Fadden T: Multination validation of anxiety, hopelessness and ineffective airway clearance, *Nursing Diagnosis* 2:57, 1991.

607. Walsh A, Walsh PA: Love, self-esteem, and multiple sclerosis, *Soc Sci Med* 29(7):793, 1989.

608. Walsh B, Rosen P: *Self-mutilation: theory, research and treatment,* New York, 1988, Guilford Press.

608a. Warbinek E, Wyness MA: Designing nursing care for patients with peripheral arterial occlusive disease. I. Update, *Cardiovasc Nurs* 22(1):1, 1986.

609. Warbinek E, Wyness MA: Designing nursing care for patients with peripheral vascular occlusive disease—Part II: nursing assessment and standard care plans, *Cardiovas Nurs* 22(2):6, 1986.

610. Warren KR, Bast RJ: Alcohol-related birth defects: an update, *Public Health Rep* 103(6):638, 1988.

610a. Weaver K: Reversible malnutrition in AIDS, *Am J Nurs* 91(9):25, 1991.

611. University of Wisconsin Hospital and Clinics: *Pulomonary rehabilitation/RESTOR services,* Madison, Wisc, 1991, University of Wisconsin.

612. Webster-Stratton C: Enhancing the effectiveness of self-administered videotape parent training for families with conduct-problem children, *J Abnorm Child Psych* 18:479, 1990.

613. Weisman AD: *On dying and denying,* New York, 1982, Behavioral Publications.

614. Weitzman J: Engaging the severely dysfunctional family in treatment: basic considerations, *Fam Process* 24:473, 1985.

615. Welch D: Anticipatory grief reactions in family members of adult patients, *Issues Ment Health Nurs* 4(2):149, 1982.

616. Welkowitz LA and others: Cognitive-behavior therapy for panic disorder delivered by psychopharmacologically oriented clinicians, *J Nerv Ment Dis* 179(8):473, 1991.

617. West JB: Pulmonary pathophysiology—the essentials, ed 3, Baltimore, 1987, Williams & Wilkins

618. Westfall U: Methods for assessing compliance, *Top Clin Nurs* 7(4):23, 1986.

619. Wewers ME, Lowe NK: A critical review of visual analogue scales in the measurement of clinical phenomena, *RINAH* 13:227, 1990.

620. Whipple B: Methods of pain control: review of research and literature, *Image J Nurs Sch* 19(3):142, 1987.

621. Whisman MA and others: Cognitive therapy with depressed inpatients: special effects on dysfunctional cognitions, *J Consult Clin Psychol* 59(2):282, 1991.

622. Whitley GG: Anxiety: defining the diagnosis, *J Psychosoc Nurs Ment Health Serv* 27(10):7, 1989.

623. Wild L: Cardiovascular problems. In Carnevali DL, Patrick M, eds: *Nursing management for the elderly,* ed 2, Philadelphia, 1986, JB Lippincott.

624. Wilkie DJ and others: Use of the McGill Pain Questionnaire to measure pain: a metaanalysis, *Nurs Res* 39(1):36, 1990.

625. Wilks SO, Meier PP: Helping mothers express milk suitable for preterm and high-risk infant feeding, *MCN* 13:121, 1988.

626. Williams JM, Long CJ, eds: *The rehabilitation of cognitive disabilities,* New York, 1987, Plenum Press.

627. Williams RL, Jackson D: Problems with sleep, *Heart Lung* 11(3):262, 1982.

628. Williams SR: *Nutrition and diet therapy,* ed 6, St Louis, 1989, Mosby–Year Book.

629. Wistrom D: Role playing, *J Psychosoc Nurs* 25(6):21, 1987.

630. Wong J and others: Effects of an experimental program on post-hospital adjustment of early discharged patients, *Int J Nurs Stud* 27(1):7, 1990.

631. Woods NF, Yates BC, Primomo J: Supporting families during chronic illness, *Image J Nurs Sch* 21(1):46, 1989.

632. Woolridge M, Fisher C: Colic, "overfeeding," and symptoms of lactose malabsorption in the breast-fed baby: a possible artifact of feed management? *Lancet* 2(8607):382, 1988.

633. Worden JW: *Grief counseling and grief therapy,* ed 2, New York, 1991, Springer.

634. Wound Care Update '91, *Nursing* 21(4):47, 1991.

635. Wright IH, Thase ME, Beck AT, eds: *The cognitive milieu: inpatient application of cognitive therapy,* New York, 1992, Guilford Press.

636. Wyness MA: Perceptual dysfunction: nursing assessment and management, *J Neurosurg Nurs* 17:105, 1985.

637. Yen PK: Eat right to avoid pressure ulcers, *Geriatr Nurs* 11(5):255, 1990.

638. Yodofsky S and others: The overt aggression scale for the objective rating of verbal and physical aggression, *Am J Psychiatry* 143:35, 1986.

639. Young JR, Terwoord BA: Stasis ulcer treatment with compression dressing, *Cleve Clin J Med* 57(6):529, 1990.

640. Zell S, Kurtz K: Severe exposure hypothermia: a resuscitation protocol, *Ann Emerg Med* 14(4):339, 1985.

641. Zerhusen JD, Boyle K, Wilson W: Out of the darkness: group cognitive therapy for depressed elderly, *J Psychosoc Nurs Ment Health Serv* 29(9):16, 1991.

642. Ziegler CC: Systemic lupus erythematosus and systemic sclerosis, *Nurs Clin North Am* 19:673, 1984.

BIBLIOGRAPHY

NANDA proceedings

Gebbie KM, Lavin MA, eds: *Classification of nursing diagnoses: proceedings of the first national conference,* St Louis, 1975, Mosby–Year Book.

Gebbie KM, ed: *Classification of nursing diagnoses: summary of the second national conference,* St Louis, 1976, Clearinghouse.

Kim MJ, Moritz DA, eds: *Classification of nursing diagnoses: proceedings of the third and fourth national conferences,* St Louis, 1982, McGraw-Hill Book Co.

Kim MJ, McFarland GK, McLane AM, eds: *Classification of nursing diagnoses: proceedings of the fifth national conference,* St Louis, 1984, Mosby–Year Book.

394

Hurley ME, ed: *Classification of nursing diagnoses: proceedings of the sixth conference*, St Louis, 1986, Mosby–Year Book.

McLane A, ed: *Classification of nursing diagnoses: proceedings of the Seventh Conference, St Louis*, 1987, Mosby–Year Book.

North American Nursing Diagnosis Association: *Classification of nursing diagnoses: proceedings of the eight conference*, Philadelphia, 1989, JB Lippincott.

North American Nursing Diagosis Association: *Classification of nursing diagnosis: proceedings of the ninth conference*, Philadelphia, 1991, JB Lippincott.

POCKET GUIDE TO NURSING DIAGNOSES

(In native languages, alphabetically)

ENGLISH Kim MJ, McFarland GK, McLane AM, eds: *Pocket guide to nursing diagnoses,* ed 5, St Louis, 1993, Mosby-Year Book, Inc.

FRENCH Kim MJ, McFarland G, McLane AM: *Guide pratique des diagnostics infimiers,* ed 3, Boucherville, Québec, 1989, Gaëtan Morin Éditeur.

ITALIAN Kim MJ, McFarland GK, McLane AM: *Diagnosi infermieristiche e piani di assistenza,* ed 3, Milano, 1991, Edizioni Sorbona Milano.

SPANISH Kim MJ, McFarland GK, McLane AM: *Manual de diagnóstico en enfermeria,* ed 3, Madrid, 1990, Interamericana—McGraw-Hill.

Glossary

contextual factors Relevant and important factors that contribute to wellness diagnoses.

defining characteristics Signs and symptoms indicating the presence of a nursing diagnosis.

diagnostic label Terminology used to name/label a nursing diagnosis.

etiology Previous term for related factors.

expected outcomes Changes in patient behaviors resulting from nursing interventions.

functional health pattern Health patterns useful in assessing human functioning.

function level classification*

    0 = Completely independent.

    1 = Requires use of equipment or device.

    2 = Requires help from another person for assistance, supervision, or teaching.

    3 = Requires help from another person and equipment device.

    4 = Dependent; does not participate in activity.

life processes Events/processes occurring throughout the lifespan that are related to health status.

NANDA North American Nursing Diagnosis Association.

nursing diagnosis† A clinical judgment about an individual, family, or community responses to actual and potential health problems/life processes. Nursing diagnoses provide the basis for selection of nursing interventions to achieve outcomes for which the nurse is accountable.

patient goals/expected outcomes Goals the patient will achieve or achieve in part as a result of nursing interventions, along

---

*Code adapted from Jones E and others: *Patient classification for long-term care: users' manual*, HEW, Publication No. HRA-74-3107, November 1974.

†Approved at the Ninth Conference on Classification of Nursing Diagnoses.

with changes in patient behavior, function, cognition, and affect, indicating goal achievement.

potential nursing diagnosis Now referred to as high-risk nursing diagnosis.

related factors Factors contributing to an *actual* nursing diagnosis.

risk factors Predisposing factors that increase vulnerability to the development of a nursing diagnosis (used with *high risk* nursing diagnoses).

signs and symptoms Objective manifestations and subjective sensation, including perception and feelings.

taxonomy The science of classification (i.e., the study of the general principles of scientific classification).

taxonomy I revised-1992 NANDA taxonomy that includes nursing diagnoses newly approved at the Tenth National Conference (1992).

Classification of nursing diagnoses by human response patterns (NANDA Taxonomy I — revised)

Exchanging

Altered nutrition: more than body requirements
Altered nutrition: less than body requirements
Altered nutrition: high risk for more than body requirements
High risk for infection
High risk for altered body temperature
Hypothermia
Hyperthermia
Ineffective thermoregulation
Dysreflexia
Constipation
Perceived constipation
Colonic constipation
Diarrhea
Bowel incontinence
Altered urinary elimination
Stress incontinence
Reflex incontinence
Urge incontinence
Functional incontinence
Total incontinence
Urinary retention
Altered tissue perfusion (specify type) (renal, cerebral, cardiopulmonary, gastrointestinal, peripheral)
Fluid volume excess
Fluid volume deficit
High risk for fluid volume deficit
Decreased cardiac output

Impaired gas exchange
Ineffective airway clearance
Ineffective breathing pattern
Inability to sustain spontaneous ventilation
Dysfunctional ventilatory weaning response
High risk for injury
High risk for suffocation
High risk for poisoning
High risk for trauma
High risk for aspiration
High risk for disuse syndrome
Altered protection
Impaired tissue integrity
Altered oral mucous membrane
Impaired skin integrity
High risk for impaired skin integrity
Communicating
Impaired verbal communication
Relating
Impaired social interaction
Social isolation
Altered role performance
Altered parenting
High risk for altered parenting
Sexual dysfunction
Altered family processes
Caregiver role strain
High risk for caregiver role strain
Parental role conflict
Altered sexuality patterns
Valuing
Spiritual distress (distress of the human spirit)
Choosing
Ineffective individual coping
Impaired adjustment
Defensive coping
Ineffective denial
Ineffective family coping: disabling
Ineffective family coping: compromised
Family coping: potential for growth
Ineffective management of therapeutic regimen (individuals)
Noncompliance (specify)
Decisional conflict (specify)
Health-seeking behaviors (specify)
Moving
Impaired physical mobility
High risk for peripheral neurovascular dysfunction

Activity intolerance

Fatigue

High risk for activity intolerance

Sleep pattern disturbance

Diversional activity deficit

Impaired home maintenance management

Altered health maintenance

Feeding self-care deficit

Impaired swallowing

Ineffective breastfeeding

Interrupted breastfeeding

Effective breastfeeding

Ineffective infant feeding pattern

Bathing/hygiene self-care deficit

Dressing/grooming self-care deficit

Toileting self-care deficit

Altered growth and development

Relocation stress syndrome

Perceiving

Body image disturbance

Self-esteem disturbance

Chronic low self-esteem

Situational low self-esteem

Personal identity disturbance

Sensory/perceptual alterations (specify) (visual, auditory, kinesthetic, gustatory, tactile, olfactory)

Unilateral neglect

Hopelessness

Powerlessness

Knowing

Knowledge deficit (specify)

Altered thought processes

Feeling

Pain

Chronic pain

Dysfunctional grieving

Anticipatory grieving

High risk for violence: self-directed or directed at others

High risk for self-mutilation

Post-trauma response

Rape-trauma syndrome

Rape-trauma syndrome: compound reaction

Rape-trauma syndrome: silent reaction

Anxiety

Fear

APPENDIX B

Classification of nursing diagnoses by functional health patterns

I. Health perception—health management pattern
Altered health maintenance
Altered protection
Ineffective management of therapeutic regimen
Noncompliance (specify)
High risk for infection
High risk for injury
High risk for trauma
High risk for poisoning
High risk for suffocation
Health-seeking behaviors (specify)

II. Nutritional—metabolic pattern
Altered nutrition: high risk for more than body requirements
Altered nutrition: more than body requirements
Altered nutrition: less than body requirements
Effective breastfeeding
Ineffective breastfeeding
Interrupted breastfeeding
Ineffective infant feeding pattern
High risk for aspiration
Impaired swallowing
Altered oral mucous membrane
High risk for fluid volume deficit
Fluid volume deficit (1)
Fluid volume deficit (2)
Fluid volume excess
High risk for impaired skin integrity
Impaired skin integrity

Based on Gordon M: *Manual of nursing diagnoses, 1993-1994*, St Louis, 1993, Mosby–Year Book.

Impaired tissue integrity
High risk for altered body temperature
Ineffective thermoregulation
Hyperthermia
Hypothermia

III. Elimination pattern
Constipation
Perceived constipation
Colonic constipation
Diarrhea
Bowel incontinence
Altered patterns of urinary elimination
Functional incontinence
Reflex incontinence
Stress incontinence
Urge incontinence
Total incontinence
Urinary retention

IV. Activity—exercise pattern
High risk for activity intolerance
Dysfunctional ventilatory weaning response
Inability to sustain spontaneous ventilation
High risk for peripheral neurovascular dysfunction
Activity intolerance
Impaired physical mobility
High risk for disuse syndrome
Fatigue
Bathing/hygiene self-care deficit
Dressing/grooming self-care deficit
Feeding self-care deficit
Toileting self-care deficit
Diversional activity deficit
Impaired home maintenance management
Ineffective airway clearance
Ineffective breathing pattern
Impaired gas exchange
Decreased cardiac output
Altered (specify type) tissue perfusion (renal, cerebral, cardiopul-
monary, gastrointestinal, peripheral)
Dysreflexia
Altered growth and development

V. Sleep—rest pattern
Sleep pattern disturbance

VI. Cognitive—perceptual pattern
Pain
Chronic pain
Sensory perceptual alterations (specify) (visual, auditory, kinesthetic,
gustatory, tactile, olfactory)

Unilateral neglect
Knowledge deficit (specify)
Altered thought processes
Decisional conflict (specify)

VII. Self-perception—self-concept pattern
Fear
Anxiety
Hopelessness
Powerlessness
Body image disturbance
High risk for self-mutilation
Personal identity disturbance
Self-esteem disturbance
Chronic low self-esteem
Situational low self-esteem

VIII. Role—relationship pattern
Anticipatory grieving
Dysfunctional grieving
Altered role performance
Caregiver role strain
High risk for caregiver role strain
Social isolation
Impaired social interaction
Relocation stress syndrome
Altered family processes
High risk for altered parenting
Altered parenting
Parental role conflict
Impaired verbal communication
High risk for violence: self-directed or directed at others

IX. Sexuality—reproductive pattern
Sexual dysfunction
Altered sexuality patterns
Rape-trauma syndrome
Rape-trauma syndrome: compound reaction
Rape-trauma syndrome: silent reaction

X. Coping—stress tolerance pattern
Ineffective individual coping
Defensive coping
Ineffective denial
Impaired adjustment
Post-trauma response
Family coping: potential for growth
Ineffective family coping: compromised
Ineffective family coping: disabling

XI. Value—belief pattern
Spiritual distress (distress of the human spirit)

Index

Italic entries indicate corresponding care plans.

404

406